the Healing burnout guide

A collection of daily perspectives, reflection & artistry

Proficient

Dr. Richard C. Scepura, DNP, MBA/MHA, RN, NEA-BC, CDN

curation by nancy nixon ensign

Hard Cover ISBN: 979-8-9851198-7-9
Paperback ISBN: 979-8-9851198-8-6
Journal (B&W) ISBN: 979-8-9851198-9-3
Journal (Color) ISBN: 979-8-9860957-1-4
Workbook ISBN: 79-8-9860957-2-1
eBook ISBN: 979-8-9860957-3-8
Hybrid ISBN: 979-8-9860957-4-5

Disclaimer

Neither this nor any other book should be used as a substitute for professional medical care or treatment. It is advisable to seek the guidance of a healthcare provider before implementing any of the approaches to health suggested in this book. The book was written to provide select information to the public concerning burnout and related topics. Research in this field is ongoing and subject to interpretation. Neither the publisher, the producer, nor the author takes any responsibility for any possible consequences from any treatment, action, or application of medicine or preparation by any person reading or following the information in this book.

Dedication

For Lamby

This book was written with the memory of author, Col. Wm. Hunter, in mind. He wrote common sense inspirational books such as *Pep, Think, and Ginger Snaps* in the late 1910's when the Spanish Flu, Russian Revolution, and First World War were the backdrop. Remarkably, similar situations have occurred in 2020 with the Covid-19 Pandemic, Russian aggression with social media, and a divisive civil political landscape. *Think* was a thrift store find and was given to the author of this book as a gift decades ago. The author, Richard Scepura, acknowledges all the hard workers in the U.S.A. and other countries around the globe that may be feeling overworked, stressed, and effects of burnout. Through reading, reflecting, connecting with inspiring art, and journaling, the process of healing from burnout can begin.

Acknowledgements

This book was a labor of love and written during the last two semesters of my doctoral program while undergoing career transitioning during the coronavirus pandemic. Originally, it was a small seed idea that morphed into a more extensive project. My first thank you must be to heaven and my mother, father, and sister for the many years of nurturing and support given to me as the youngest child. The generous support of my loving father during coronavirus time period while writing this book was immense, and for that, I am forever grateful. My aunts & uncles, many cousins, and of course my doggies, *Hank, Veda, and Birdie*. I hope that I make my entire family proud in *all I do*. (I try- even though I can be a little rascal).

Next, I want to praise each and every artist who willingly volunteered to be part of this project, offering their labors of love in images for the benefit of many. If there is a particular piece that you have connected with, I hope you will find the artists' contact information in that section of the book and reach out to them to support, acknowledge, or show interest in their work. It is so important to offer recognition, and I am certain each would appreciate that very much. Their work inspired me a great deal while spending many hours researching and writing the book at the Patterson Library in Westfield, NY (*Chautauqua County*).

This brings me to a very special thank you to a dear friend of mine, Nancy Nixon Ensign, the Curator of *Octagon Gallery* and primary artist showcased in this book and covers. I have known her for over thirty years from our college days at *Rochester Institute of Technology* together. She'd offer me a lift home when needed and literally went the extra mile, beyond her own town, to make sure I got home safely. Well, after so much time of lives apart and away, reconnecting together on this project challenged us both! There were days we laughed, cried, shouted, pulled teeth, and leapt for joy. It was kismet when we each knew and agreed on an idea or work of art. Her keen curation skill made the process almost seem effortless in retrospect, and she still gives me a big heartfelt lift.

Once the art was situated, my attention became much more focused on refinement and much gratitude to our first contributing editor, Tiffany Smith. Tiffany and I spent some evenings (after already busy workdays) of a 4-month pleasant period, to ready the draft manuscripts. Without

Tiffany, the constant push and responsibility toward completing each season of the book might have been adrift. I am forever thankful for all her assistance and organizational skills, helping me keep versions of the draft manuscripts in order. I highly recommend Tiffany for your technical writing or editing needs. (See: www.tlynnseditingservice.net)

Next, how do you ever graciously thank your eighth-grade English teacher enough for volunteering during her busy schedule to read and peer-review your work so many years after graduating high school? With much gratitude, I thank Dr. Jane Blystone, Ph.D., MJE, who volunteers on the prestigious *Journalism Education Association, Inc.* (JEA) Scholastic Press Rights Committee, JEA Certification Committee, and is a JEA Mentor. I hope the book brought some joy and peace for you. After all these years, you are still mentoring me, and you are so appreciated. Thank you kindly for writing the Forward.

Another peer reviewer was the Director of my Nursing program at *Clarion and Edinboro Universities*, Dr. Meg Larson. Meg was my professor and committee chair for a completely different project during the doctoral studies, in addition to peer-reviewing this book. She is one of the most patient educators I know, and she steered me in the right direction (encouraging me to write and publish), and I am grateful to her as well. I appreciate her taking the time to digest the work, offer feedback and input. Her flexibility allowed me to challenge myself in new ways of thinking and growing. I hope she enjoyed the topics and art, as well and her time reading the book. In some small way, I hope it helped inspire her. I'm sure she had a giggle, grimace, or grin while reviewing! I thank her greatly for writing the additional Forward.

Next came the final review of the manuscript with contributing editor, Jessica Olma. Jessica came recommended to us by *Spotlight Publishing.* Jessica's editing refined the works to expand our audience. It took me a little while, but we reached the end of the final manuscript as I began writing these acknowledgments. I am forever grateful for her expertise, and professionalism. I hope the book brought insight and joy to her as well, and that the information in the book was of interest and helpful. Thank you for making the final editing phase very smooth, Jessica! Her business is at Scribe Syndicate, and I recommend her to all.

After I had the first round of peer reviewed manuscript completed, I invited other reviewers to read the books. I wanted to be certain that there was a multi-disciplinary review from professionals before going to print. Dr. Matthew Conner, MD, Dr. Deborah Cohan, MD, MPH, Dr. Preston Davis, PsyD, Josephine Poulin, MSN, APRN, FNP-C, and Dr. Patricia Boulogne, DC, CCSP, MaoM, AP, CFLP, CFMP. I am so thankful for their time, efforts, and appreciate their feedback. I also would like to thank Dr. Patricia Benner, Nurse Theorist and Author of *From Novice to Expert* for inspiring this work.

Our graphic designer for the second, third, and fourth book in the series is Tom Olson. Tom is the owner of the graphic design *Pixel-Pencil Studio* as well as the boutique publishing firm, *Morningstar Press*. Tom creates beautiful and unique graphic designs for independent authors. He offers a comprehensive and flexible array of services. Tom took the design of the second book in our series to an evolved level and even further with the third book, *Proficient* and we are very grateful for his expertise. I look forward to what he does with *Expert*, our fourth book (as well as my next book series which is half-written at this time- more to come on that!). Working with Tom is such a pleasure, he is professional, organized, creative, and very timely. I would highly recommend Tom and his businesses, which offers authors creative book design as well as knowledgeable and practical guidance to take their book project from the idea phase to a virtual book launch – making their projects come to life. Thank you so much, Tom!

With that, last but not least, are the many other friends, colleagues, and loved ones along the way in my life that have been supportive, not just during this period of creating the book, but faithfully through thick and thin. They know who they are: Doreen, Liza, Vicki, Mary Jane S., Audra, Nate, Alain, Mary Jo, Sharin, David, Jason, Douglas, Jimmy, Avi, Ian, my next-door neighbors Nicholas, Tiffany, and Rosie. Dawn and Nicholas & Brandon, Elizabeth G, Michael V., Nurse Joy, Heidi (my teacher of *Nadi Shodhana Pranayama*), Preston, Daphne, Maria, Phil, Libby O., the entire Boston *Eclipse* crew including Brenda, David, Cyndi, Bob, Steve, Paul, Marianne, Denise, Boston's North End *La Summa* Barbara and Siobhan from *Pomodoro*, through the years (forever grateful for beautiful memories), my North End friends David Archer, Billy, Desi, Chip, and hometown friends Lisa Conti, Julie & Randy (always missed), Lisa Monte, Ruthie and Jan, Toni & JT, Uncle Clay, the Clines, Dunster Street Pat and Scottie, my *Maui Ohana*- Kelly, Erina, Uncle Brett, Dale and April, my special JP 39-bus friend, Peeps, Dr. Paula Sperry (talk radio host at *WOMR Provincetown*), the countless friends and neighbors that inspired me over decades in Provincetown in the East End and West End, St. Elizabeth's, BIDMC, Mass General and Seattle Children's dialysis nurses, and countless others (those I may have missed acknowledging due to my humanness). To all my professors and *alma maters* RIT, UMASS Boston, Pfeiffer U., and Clarion and Edinboro Universities- *Thank you, thank you.*

Preface

Considerable improvements in clinical work and learning environments in every healthcare setting must be prioritized for all disciplines to prevent and mitigate clinician burnout and foster wellbeing for the overall health of medical professionals, patients, and the nation. According to *The National Academies of Sciences, Engineering, & Medicine* (2019), "between 35 and 54 percent of U.S. nurses and physicians experience burnout symptoms, along with 45 to 60 percent of medical students and residents." Many studies have indicated burnout to be a common problem among all clinical disciplines and across care settings.[1]

Studies conducted in 2020 have shown further evidence of the rising burnout. One study known as the *Physicians' Foundation/Merritt Hawkins Study* concluded that about 55 percent of healthcare workers described their job as negative due to the conditions. The *Medscape* study revealed that physician burnout has increased by 2 percent since 2018. *The AMN Healthcare* biennial nursing study revealed that a rising 63 percent of nurses reported burnout and 44 percent often wanted to quit as a result.[2]

Making matters even more serious, the start of 2020 introduced our world to the pandemic known as COVID-19 (coronavirus 2019), which no one was prepared to handle. Stress, anxiety, and burnout among healthcare workers during the outbreak reached an all-time high due to the fear of catching the virus and spreading it to others, as well as the uncertainty of how the outbreak would affect us overall both socially and economically. The only option for healthcare workers to make it through this time period is/was to remain hopeful and look for opportunities to practice self-care, professional advocacy, celebrate successes, and find time to take breaks from stress. It is imperative for employers to encourage their employees to practice acts of self-care in an attempt to reduce stress and burnout.[3] These are alarming statistics of burnout in healthcare workers. Imagine what other industries may have similar situations.

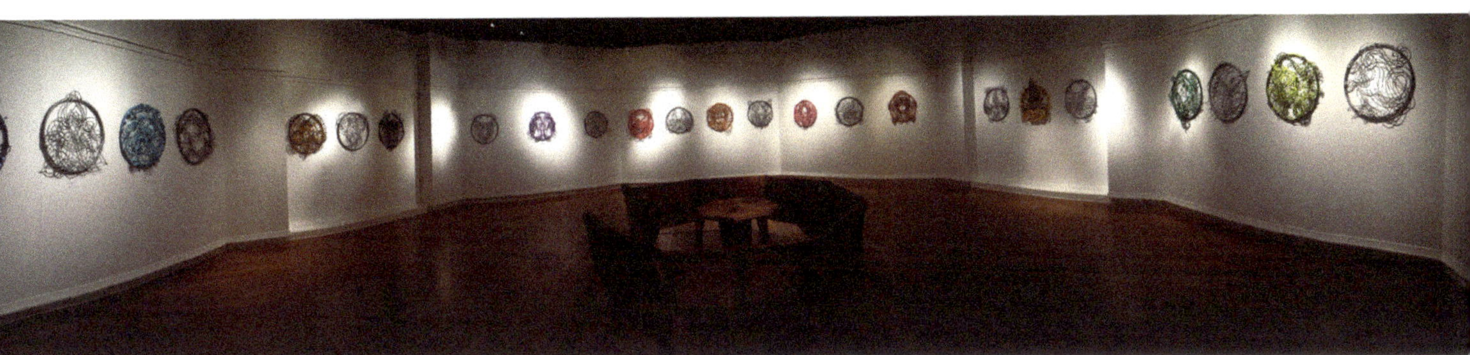

Jon Chisholm in Octagon Gallery

The Octagon Gallery is part of the world-famous Patterson Library in Westfield, NY (Chautauqua County) and hosts several artists for monthly exhibitions in a variety of mediums.

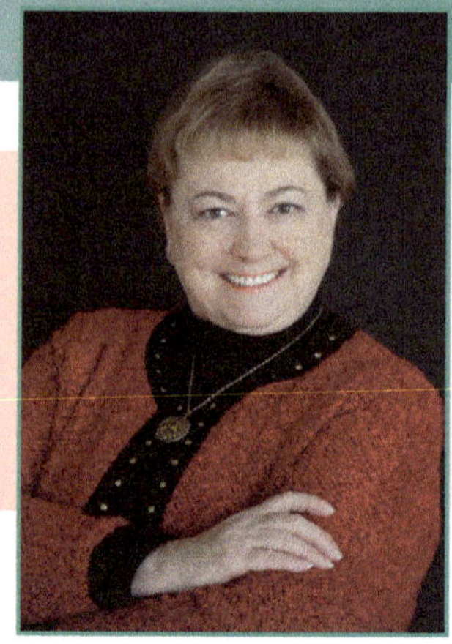

In a time of great stress for many, this pandemic has moved many professionals in healthcare, education, and other essential services into burnout mode. In this 365-day self-reflection journal Richard has prepared, the reader will practice strong reflective thinking that provides a researched approach to reduce stress, and concerning day-to-day frustrations that lead to burnout. Richard has always been an empathetic person. I first met him when he joined my yearbook staff in high school. As his teacher, I watched his great love for helping people. As he graduated and followed a career path in healthcare as a nurse, I was so impressed that he continued to be a helper and empathetic individual. His career has led him to be a traveling nurse, nurse manager, director, consultant, and continue his education at both the graduate and doctoral levels.

Richard has seen and helped deal with burnout in his profession. We have talked about this for some time and I am so pleased to see this book emerge as a tool for individuals who work with many patients, clients, students, customers on any given day to deal with the stress of caring for others. This reflection journal is the outworking of his skill in caring for other nurses, healthcare professionals, and the public. It is a much needed reflective tool for anyone in our time. Each season of this self-reflection journal gives the reader the option of reflecting in writing and/or in thoughtful self-reflection about ways to calm the mind and heart. The art he has selected also provides beautiful aesthetic experiences for the reader. Professionals who feel stationary in their careers will find this journal a perfect way to articulate goals for future advancement and to develop self-confidence.

It is my great pleasure to recommend this book to you as I have read every word and experienced the uplifting nature of these daily reflection exercises Richard has presented in this journaling workbook.

Enjoy,

Jane Blystone, PhD, MJE
JEA Mentor Program Chair
JEA Certification Committee
PA School Press Association Board of Directors

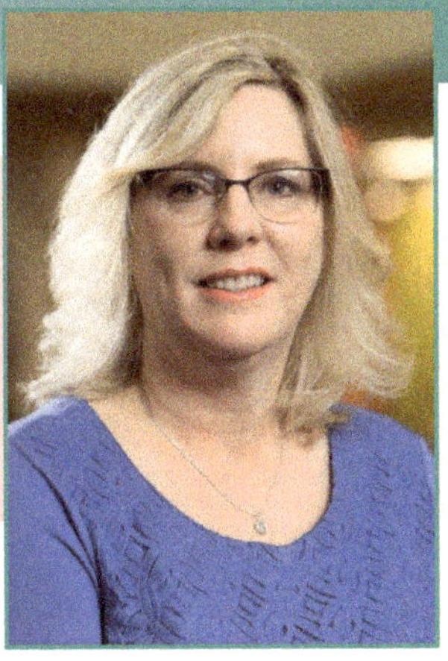

In living memory, there has never been a time WITH SO MANY EVENTS that have touched SO MANY PEOPLE across all walks of life. In normal times, professionals in some careers face high burnout rates. This is, of course, exacerbated by the global pandemic, which strains them professionally, and, in many cases, personally.

We all hope that we have a period of healing coming soon. The world's trauma is largely beyond any individual control, which can lead to increased feelings of pain, disempowerment, and burnout. This self-reflection journal is a wonderful resource that allows readers to spend as much or as little time as they have and still make an impact on their mental health and carry on in their essential careers.

This book is written by Dr. Richard Scepura, who has authentic experience in burnout, its consequences, and solutions to improve higher functioning at work, and more importantly, higher quality of life. His unique view of the problems we face and the solutions we have at our disposal make it a must-read for this time. It is also a resource that, like many good reads, can be re-read and continue to offer new significance to the reader as their circumstances change. This makes it an excellent addition to any library and a good gift idea for students entering the workplace, schools, or new professions in our changing world.

Dr. Meg Larson, DNP, FNP-C
Primary Care Provider
Veterans Health Associate Professor, Edinboro University

Introduction

There is a body of evidence that explains burnout as a very real global phenomenon experienced by many people in different fields in the workforce. The numbers of those experiencing burnout are increasing despite the knowledge. "Like a frog jumping into a boiling pot of water," all at once, you may feel the effects of burnout because it may not have been evident to you along the way. But it doesn't just happen all at once. It is similar to a slow-moving python that grips its prey, and with an insidious, gradual hold, it squeezes the living daylights out of you.

The emotional, spiritual, physical, psychological, and educational dimensions of a person are impacted greatly when they experience burnout. Each dimension needs special attention to achieve the self-care that is siphoned from you when burnout occurs, often leaving you feeling powerless. In this delightful and impactful book series I created for you, *The Healing Burnout Guide,* I am inviting you, dear reader, to self-reflect. While burnout is often regarded as happening in the workplace, it may occur in your home as well.

Are you feeling stressed or fatigued from the pandemic? Are you feeling the weight of work overload and the pressure of documentation demand? Are you thinking technology has impacted how you live and work and are unhappy with the many changes? Are you becoming frustrated easily? Do you feel as if your personal and work mission are in conflict? Are you experiencing an ethical dilemma or any moral distress? Has it reached a tipping point where you feel like your compassion and service to others seems insincere, and you just go through the motions of performing tasks at your job? Have you become cynical or depersonalized in your approach with people? If so, then I think this book series will really help you.

In my role as a nurse leader, I have witnessed many employees suffering from the effects of burnout. The benefits of performing self-reflection on the variety of topics included will help you expand your emotional quotient (EQ). You will learn how to set limits and put burnout prevention front and center in your mind. As we meander together, exploring and absorbing perspectives, responding to self-reflection questioning, inspired by artistry, you will truly begin to heal on your workbook journey. Give yourself the time to journal daily. **Do not wait!** I promise the benefits of this journaling book will help you immensely to stave off burnout by learning to improve your self-care strategies. My best wishes as you proceed to make self-care your number one priority.

SEASON THREE

Proficient

JULY 1

Day 182

My Hobbies

Rates of burnout amid doctors in the U.S. are currently at their highest. Physician burnout levels are also significantly higher than the mainstream population. The satisfaction of physicians' life-work balance continues to decrease. Finding hobbies, such as painting, fishing, playing an instrument, or knitting, can be helpful. Also, doing crafts or exploring the great outdoors can help you unwind. Hobbies are a productive way of coping with stress management and recuperating from a demanding professional life.[194]

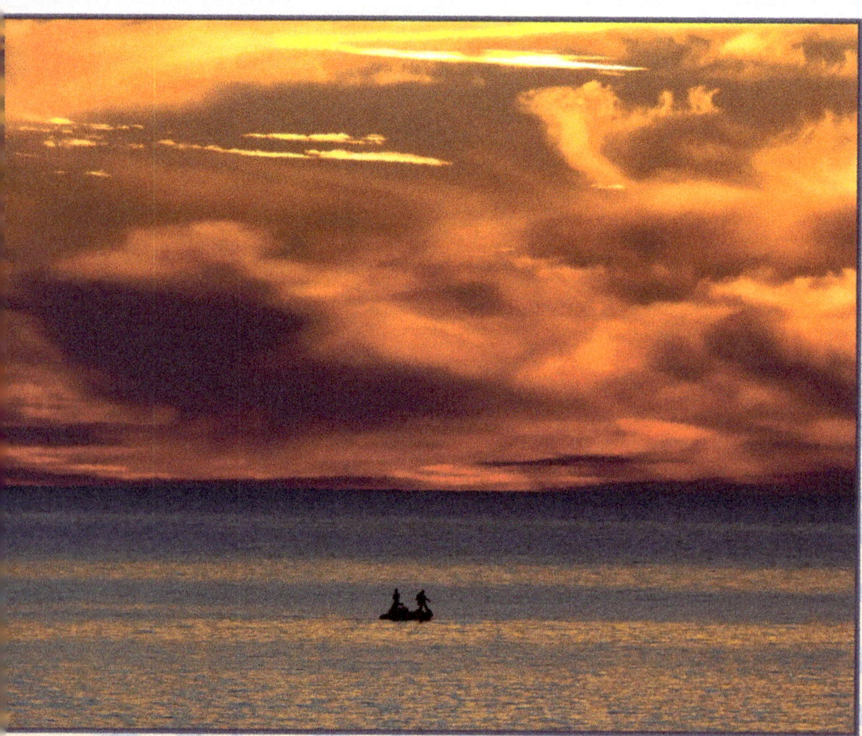

Courtesy of Spar Ki

Today I will consider my hobbies. Is it time to take up a new one? Managing stress is very important and having an outlet is a great way to expel energy in a positive way. How can you work your hobby into an already overburdened schedule? What hobbies interest you that could help you create a better work-life balance? Write about your answers in your journal.

JULY 2

Day 183

Patience

Some signs of burning out include a lack of patience, creativity, enthusiasm, and imagination in your daily routine. Burnout can bring you to the brink of sanity. You may feel as if you can no longer give, have sapped energy, and tested emotions to the depth of your core.[195]

Today I will think about my patience. Are you out of it? If so, what is your plan to replenish the empty cup? It can be time for self-care activities if your mood is short and you are out of patience with everything and everyone. Use your imagination – what creative talents are being brought to the surface? Journal about your level of patience. Write about all the self-care activities you have been doing so far this year. It takes patience and enthusiasm to achieve your goals.

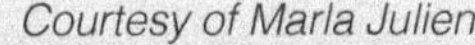

Courtesy of Marla Julien

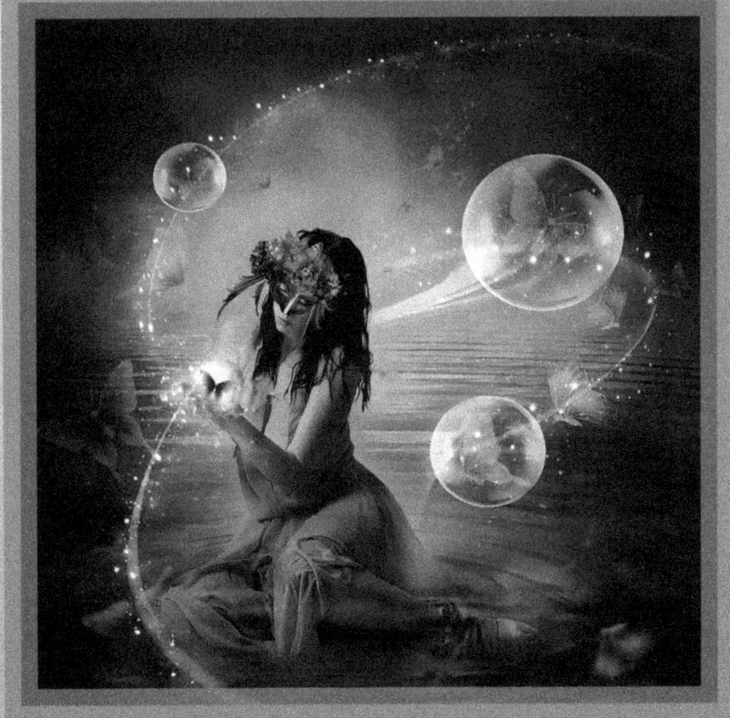

JULY 3

Day 184

Practice Makes Perfect

Courtesy of Edward Berkise

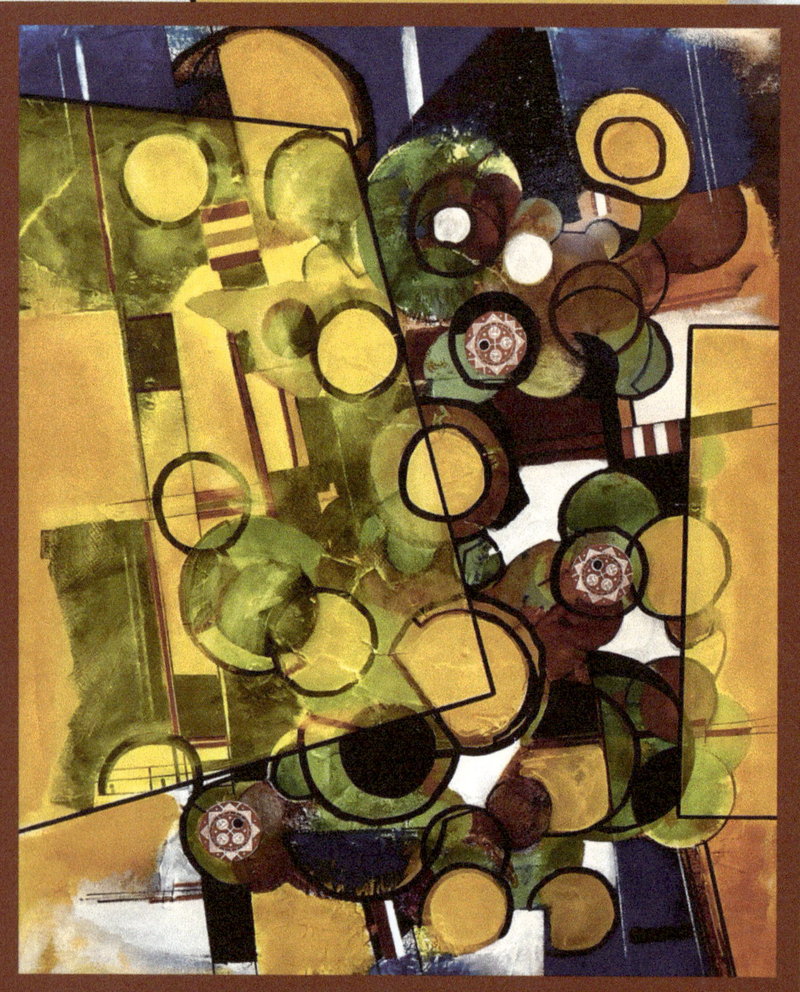

The process to make long-lasting change frequently demands attempting new and different things. It could be walking a new route to work to avoid a troublesome location. Perhaps it's practicing new ways of coping with or facing old challenges. Or reaching for others to help when you would usually do something alone. Practice makes perfect when achieving a set of new behaviors. You may notice that when you get better at making changes, odds increase for success when it matters most. As you continue practicing, old habits get replaced with newer ones.[196]

Today I will think about something I want to practice and perfect. You can begin something new and practice as much as you want. Become proficient by letting yourself try. Journal about three things you would like to practice and perfect now. Remember, when you learn new things, it can be a great strategy for defeating burnout.

Independence

Independence is when people feel free to express themselves when learning, experiencing, and improving daily living. It is seen as a satisfying desire to become a more secure person without disconnecting from personal values. Independence is a form of originality that empowers people to speak their minds and free themselves from ignorance. Many view autonomy as a means of living the most fulfilling life, being bolder and stronger each day. For many, this sense of freedom can be about a life pursuit or fulfilling peaceful ventures. The responsibility of independence can be terrifying since being free to make our own choices also requires taking responsibility for the consequences. Your life is a painting. You can choose which colors to paint with, exactly as you wish.[197]

Today I will reflect on my independence. What does it mean to you? Does independence allow you to practice acts of self-care? Are you aware that although you are free to make your own choices, your actions have consequences? Do you often speak your mind? Do you live life to the fullest? Do you feel you have too little, enough, or too much independence? Write about your feelings of freedom in your journal.

Courtesy of Ann Parker

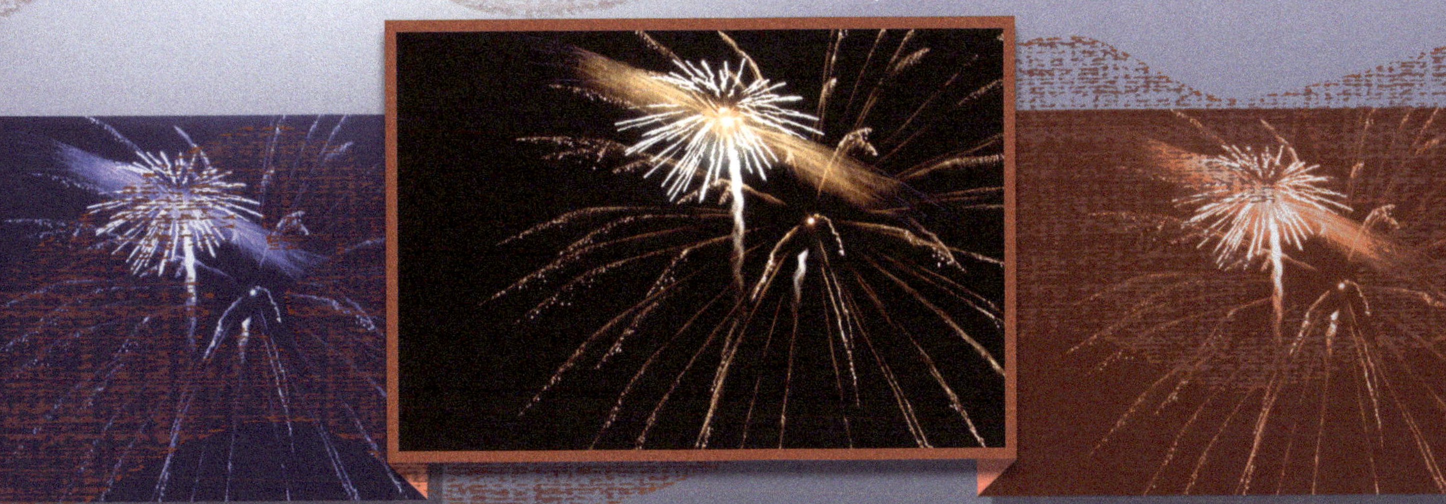

Not Getting What You Want

Day 186

When you're not getting what you want, it can trigger emotions that you will need to manage. This can be good! You will have to locate new solutions to old challenges. This is also good! You may have to totally abort a plan that doesn't work, begin a new strategy, or abandon a dream. This is very painful but creates growth. Don't sugarcoat the problem. Not getting what you want is painful. It hurts and causes a spiraling question of self-worth. We may be tossed into ruminating on whether we'll survive the pain.[198]

Today I will remember that I can't always get what I want. It doesn't feel good to sacrifice what you want all the time. Wait a day, week, month, or year and see how things evolve. Sometimes what you wanted wasn't worth having. There may be another destination that lies ahead. Be patient, don't stress, and it will come. Journal about a time you couldn't get something you really wanted. Did you later discover whether it was worth having or not? Did you eventually get over the pain? Did you discover a new and better path?

Courtesy of Patti Larson

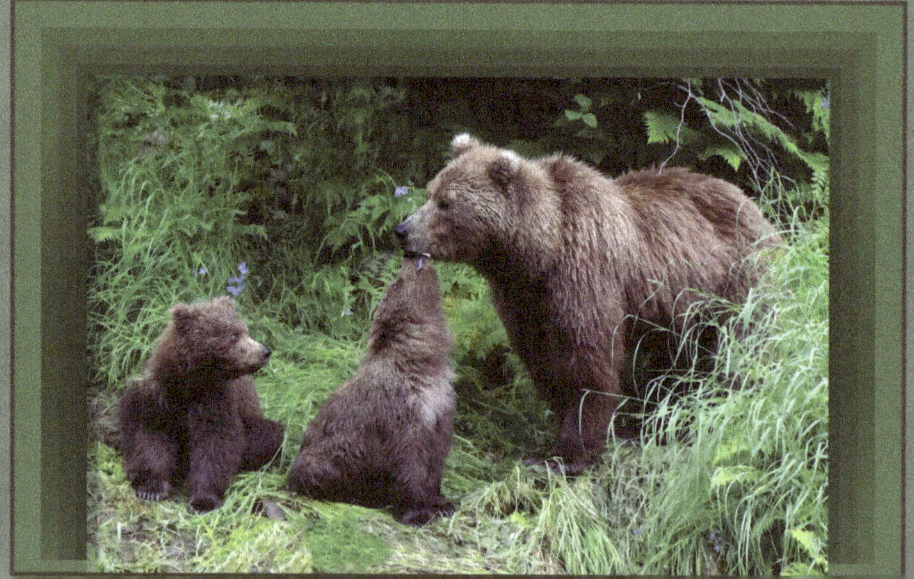

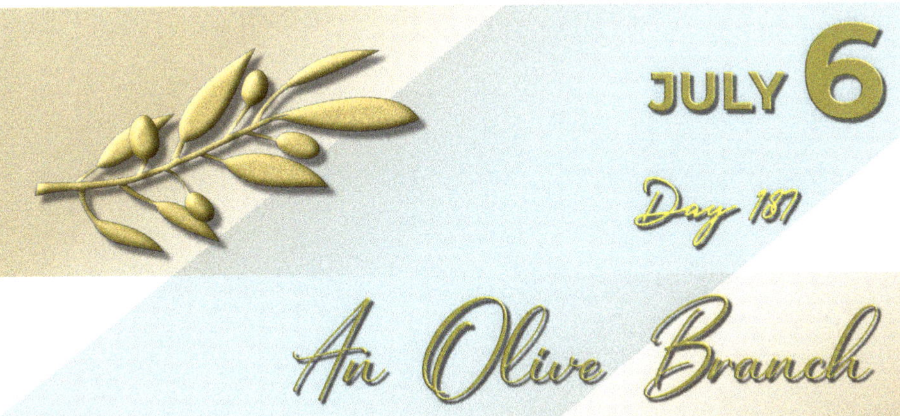

JULY 6

Day 187

An Olive Branch

As early as the ancient Greeks and Romans, the olive branch has been a symbol of peace. Extending an olive branch today is commonly thought of as making an agreement between two parties at odds. It is interesting that something so delicate can carry the burden of humanity's most substantial gift - forgiveness. Forgiving someone is a crucial element of peace. Think about achieving peace with a person that you are holding a grudge against.[199]

Today I will consider a grudge I am holding. Try extending an olive branch and forgive. Let go of the hard feelings which are so stressful and only harm your inner peace. You don't have to forget what happened; just try to set it aside and let go of feelings of anger and disappointment. Journal about a time when you extended an olive branch to someone. Did you feel more at peace once you allowed yourself to forgive and move on? Has anyone ever extended an olive branch to you?

Courtesy of Mara Rubin

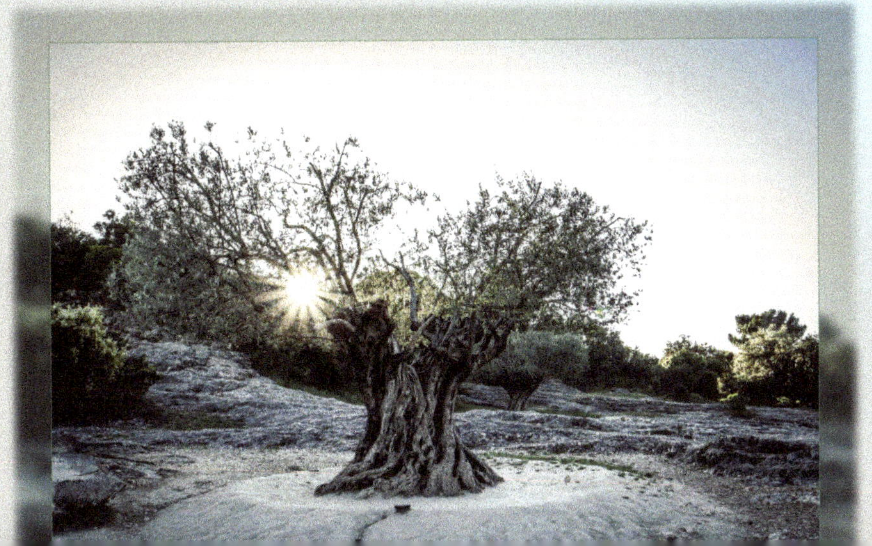

JULY 7

Day 188

Recognition

Courtesy of Rebecca Samler

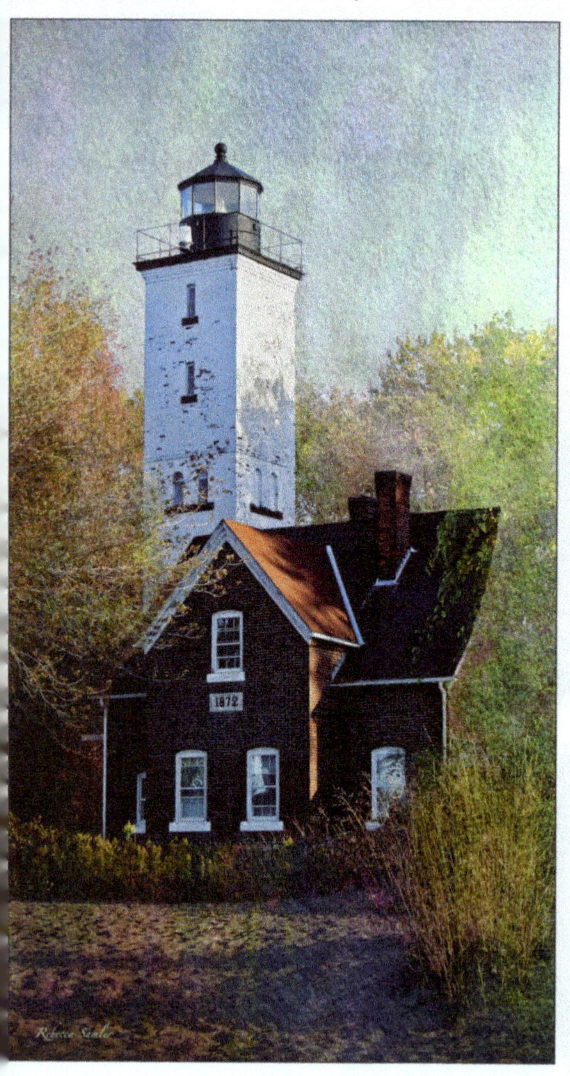

There is a golden rule in the office, "recognize others as you would like to be recognized." It is important to appreciate people for working hard and make sure they receive the recognition and rewards they deserve. It is the kindest way to do things. It assists in building necessary relationships with coworkers. How does this help you receive the recognition you deserve at work? Recognizing others inspires them to display a similar attitude of appreciation toward you. When you acknowledge others, it increases the probability that they will do the same.[200]

Today I will think about recognizing others for their good work. I will intentionally look for opportunities to be thankful for them. I will also think about my own recognition. Are you the type of person that doesn't necessarily need or desire to be publicly recognized, or do you like it? Not everyone does, so be sensitive towards people and their individual feelings about public recognition. For some, a note or certificate of appreciation may mean more. Write about your thoughts concerning recognition in your journal.

JULY 8

Day 189

Prudence

Prudence means to be cautious about the choices you make and to stop and think before you act. It is known as the power of restraint. When being prudent, you will be sure to avoid risks. You are cautious about doing or saying something that is regrettable later.[201]

Today I will reflect on prudence. Think about the choices that you have made and whether they have been prudent to your wellbeing. Consider the risks you have taken and the things you have said and done. If you are not entirely happy with those choices, journal about your plan going forward and being more prudent. Maybe you've made wise choices and have successfully avoided risk. It can be stressful to find yourself in a place of regret.

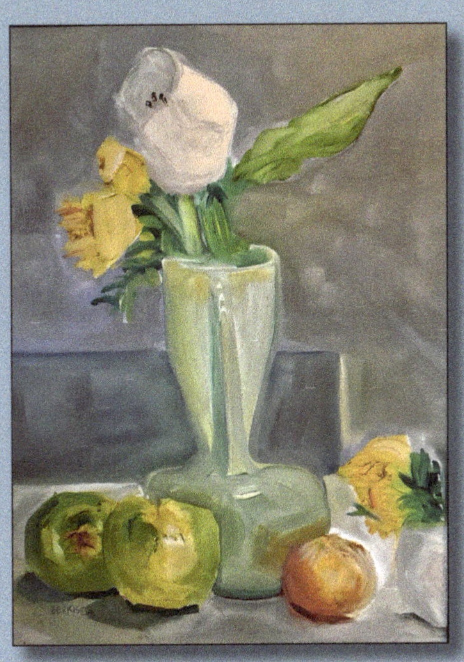

Courtesy of Edward Berkise

JULY 9

Day 190

Economic Insecurity

The 2016 Work and WellBeing Survey by the American Psychological Association reported that more than a third of working adults in the United States complain that job insecurity is a notable source of their stress. Sadly, research has proven that job uncertainty leads to negative, substantial, and pervasive outcomes. For instance, workers who feel they may lose their jobs are more apt to report feelings of burnout, decreased organizational commitment, and lower work engagement than job-secure peers.[202]

Today I will realize the startling statistic that 33.3% of adult working Americans report job insecurity and that this is stressful and significant to so many. Being thankful if you have a job is a great way to begin the day. When a person feels insecure about their economic situation, their commitment and engagement shrink. Evaluate and describe in your journal whether you feel secure in your job, and if not, is there a plan you can make?

Courtesy of Umberto Kamperveen

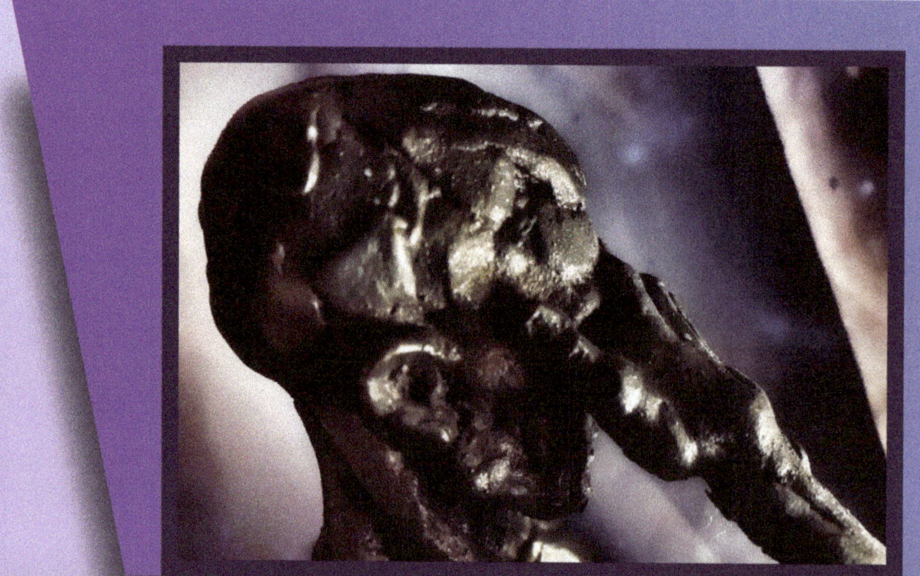

Life Isn't Always Easy

It is often difficult for people to realize the level of responsibility needed for serving others while maintaining a spirit of understanding and sensitivity. It is also important to support mutual consideration and trust while preserving the highest morals and standards. Making an impact in another person's life isn't simple or pretty. It takes a special someone to recognize the impact they can have on others, especially when things aren't perfect.[203]

Today I will realize that life isn't always easy, especially getting up very early in the morning and being your best self while wearing a smile each day at work. Give yourself some credit and recognize that it isn't easy to perform under the stressful situations happening around you. Nurture yourself today and pat yourself on the back for the good work you do. There may not be anyone to recognize you in the workplace as you deserve. Journal about a time when things weren't perfect, but you made the best of it anyway. Give examples of how you made an impact on others' lives.

Courtesy of Linda Probst

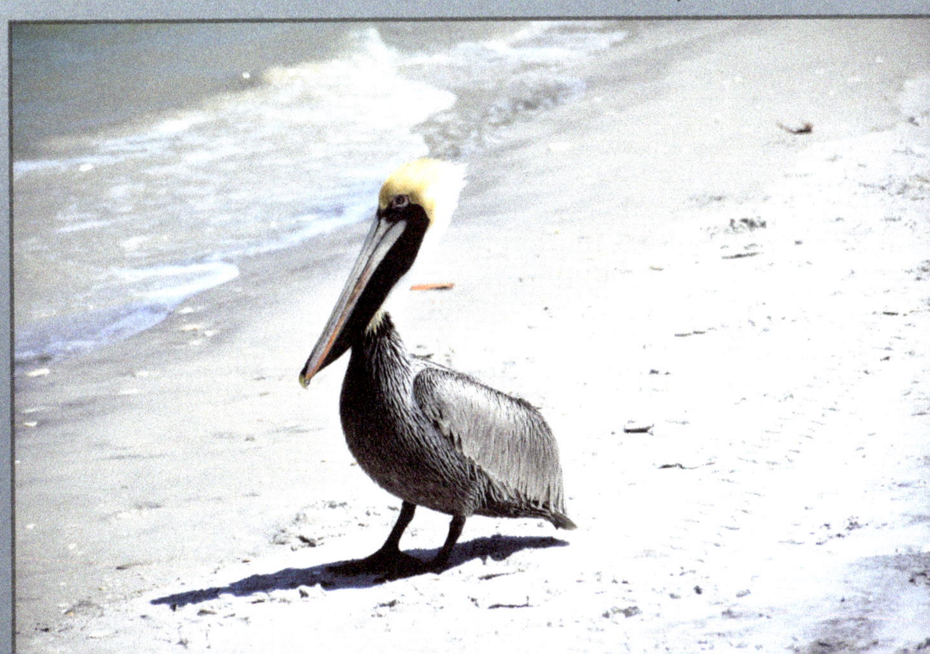

JULY 11

Day 192

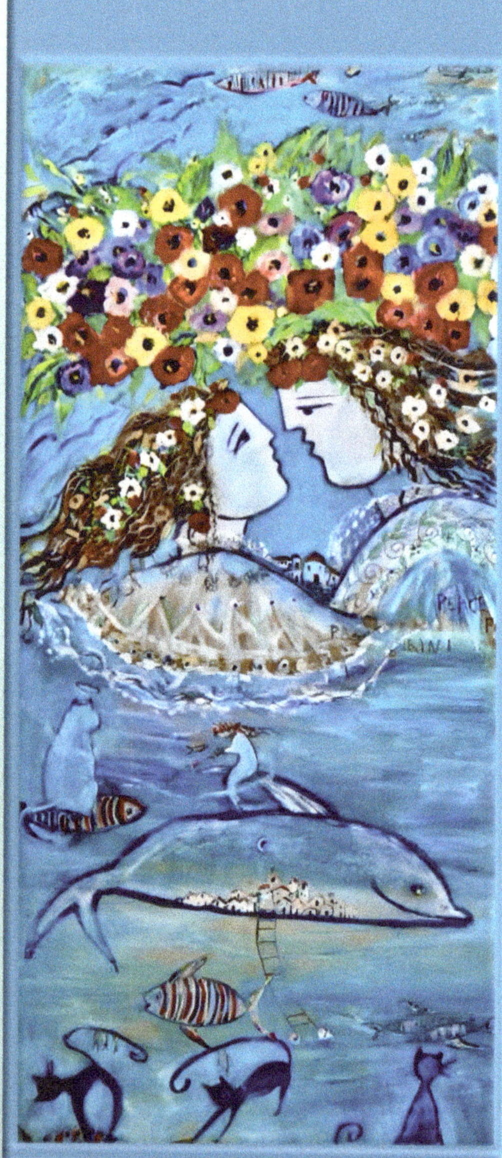

Courtesy of Maika Gonzalez

Feeling Appreciated

When you genuinely feel appreciated, it's uplifting. Basically, appreciation gives us a sense of safety, which allows us to perform at our best level for work. It can also be energizing. When we feel that our value is at risk, and often it is, we become preoccupied with worry. Fretting diverts and drains us of the energy needed to create value.[204]

Today I will make an active effort to appreciate others around me. Journal about how you can tell others how much their work contributes to the mission and that you are glad they are part of the team. What are some things that you could say to them? Something as simple as appreciating another coworker first thing in the morning can set the tone for the entire day and create a less stressful environment. Try it.

JULY 12

Day 193

Stop Worrying

Try to reflect on your troubles in different ways. You might feel as though your worries are derived from external factors such as other people, stressful events, or facing tough circumstances. However, continuing to worry about it is self-imposed stress. The triggers may come from outside sources, but internal running dialogues are what preserve the actual anxiety. When you can let go of the notion that worrying is somehow helping, you are able to handle your anxiety and stress in better, effective ways.[205]

Today I will acknowledge that external stressors may trip my trigger and make my anxiety level rise exponentially. However, healthy self-talk is what gets me through. In your journal, try brainstorming about how you can stop the ruminations and unnecessary worry. Instead, think about how worry harms you. What things can you try to let go of worry? Perhaps, try going for a long walk outside or watching the sunset today.

Courtesy of Patti Larson

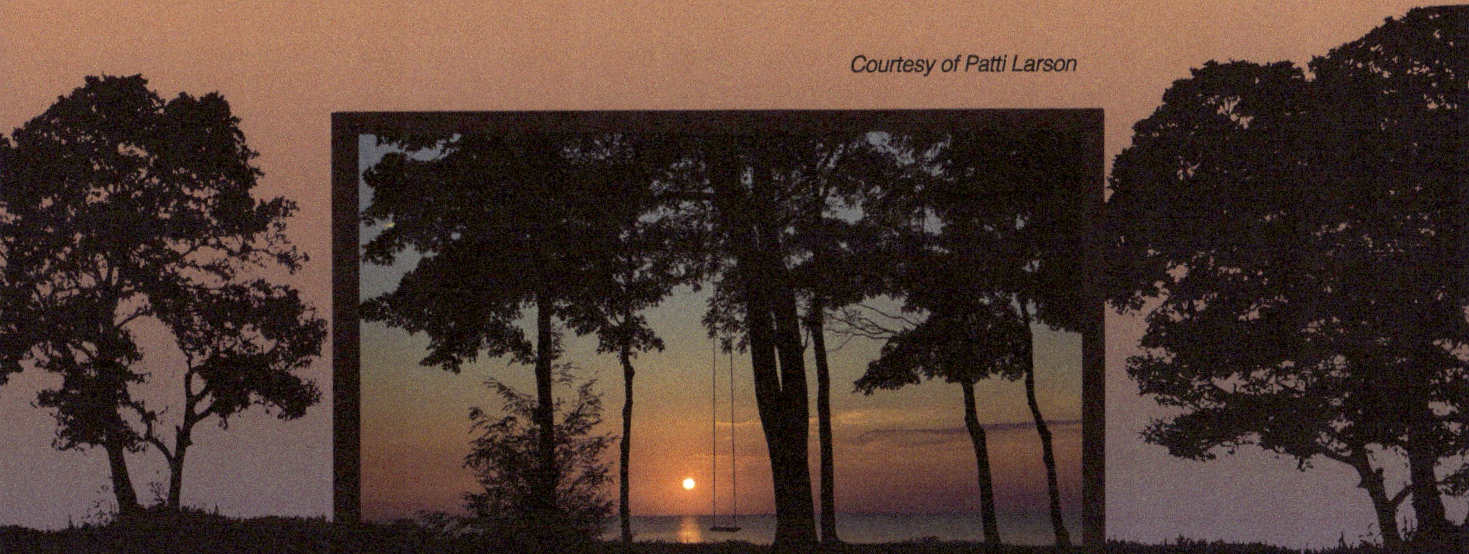

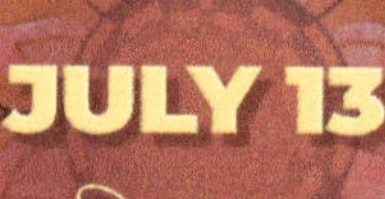

I'm Worth It

Having happiness and success in your life starts with understanding your value and worth. To feel truly alive, you must obtain a powerful sense of confidence and self-worth. When you genuinely have faith in yourself, you'll become more effective and efficient throughout every aspect of your life. Your self-esteem will increase, allowing you to recognize the difference you can make. Become clear, know your morals, engage in more fulfilling activities, and say, "I'm worth it." [206]

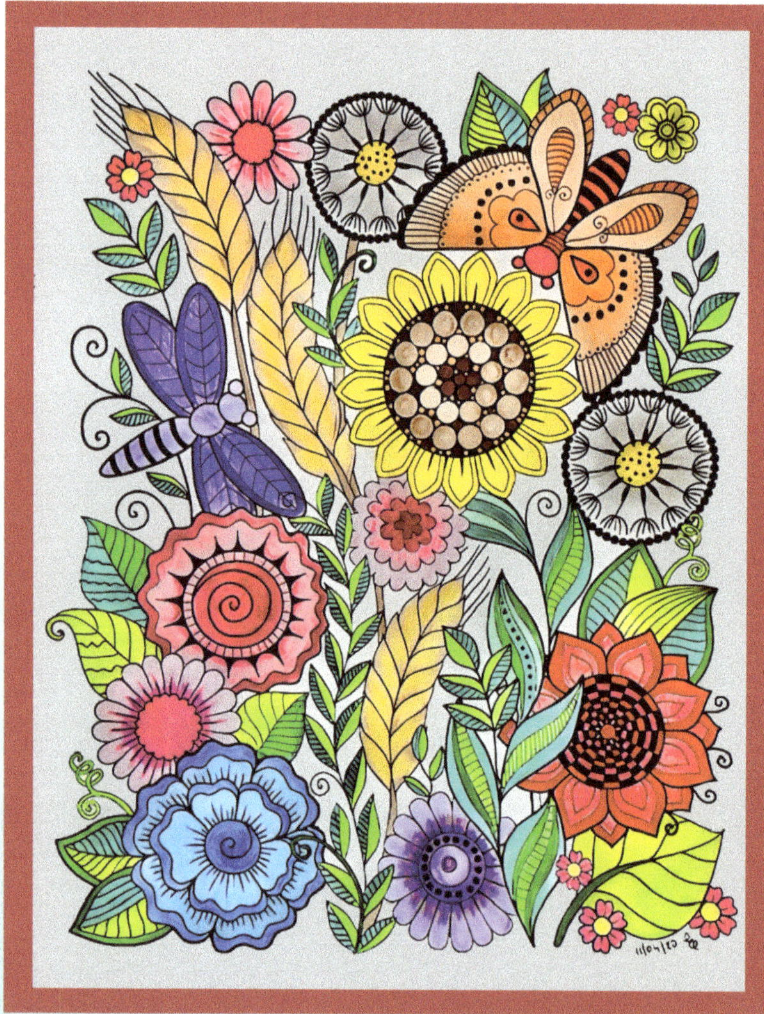

Courtesy of Eduardo Andres

Today I will consider how I think or feel about my own value. Do you have a positive attitude about the value you deliver and confidence that the work you do matters? Believe in yourself no matter how others may try to devalue you. The only person that can bring you down is yourself. Tell yourself that you are worth it, and you know it. Journal about a time when you had to recognize your own worth to make a difference in your life. Do others validate your worth?

JULY 14

Day 195

Pay and Economics

Inequality of income in the U.S. has become more dramatic. For instance, a chief executive officer is paid over 380 times the typical salary of a standard employee. If your income seems to be shrinking instead of growing, it isn't just you and your employer; it's a national problem. Private companies, large-scale nonprofits, and the public sector are seeing consumer purchasing power being sapped, undermining the American middle class, and harming our economy.[207]

Today I will realize that I may not be receiving fair pay for the work I do. It isn't your imagination. Income inequality is a very real problem in the United States. The shrinking middle class is harmful. Not having enough income causes stress and adds to the factors that contribute to burnout in the workplace. Journal about your concerns with fair pay within your workplace. Is your leadership doing anything to try and address those concerns? What are your thoughts about stinginess, pay, and economics?

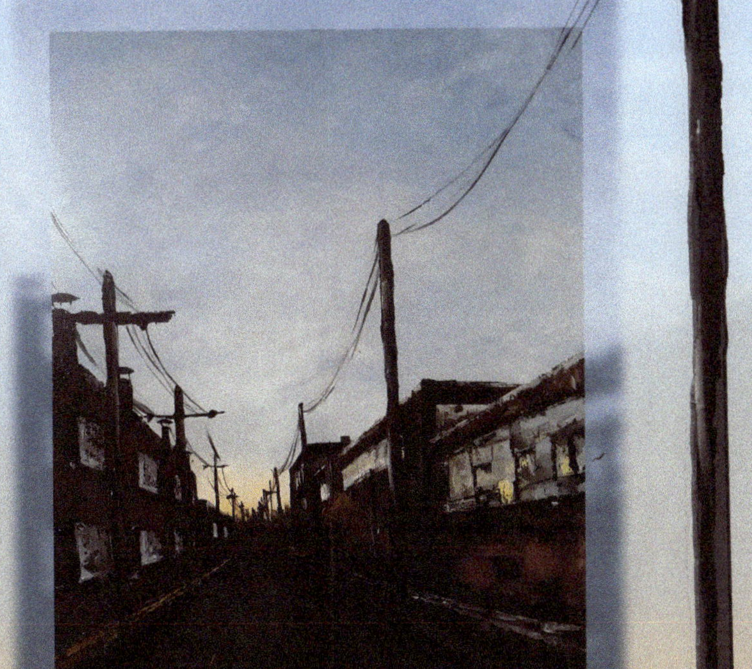

Courtesy of Susan Gutierrez

JULY 15 *Day 196*

Sharing Your Stories

Realize that your voice matters - your stories matter. We see now, better than ever, how important it is to use our voice, share our stories, and learn from one another. Real-life lessons are the best experiences. Stories often elicit empathy. Empathy creates caring. Caring motivates action.[208]

Today I will consider the stories I share. When you tell your stories, you are giving yourself a voice and validation, and you are teaching others about things that happened. Your stories can help others learn. Leadership arises from the ability to share stories and engage others. Journal about three stories that are important to you and have them readily available to share with others. What lessons do your stories tell? Do they create empathy, caring, and motivate actions?

Courtesy of Maika Gonzalez

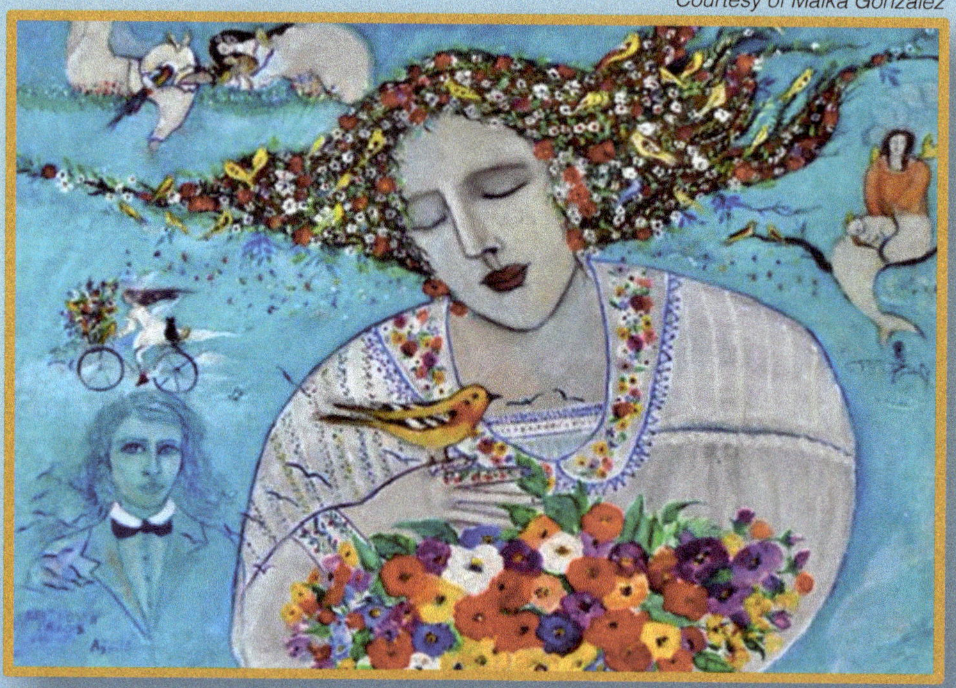

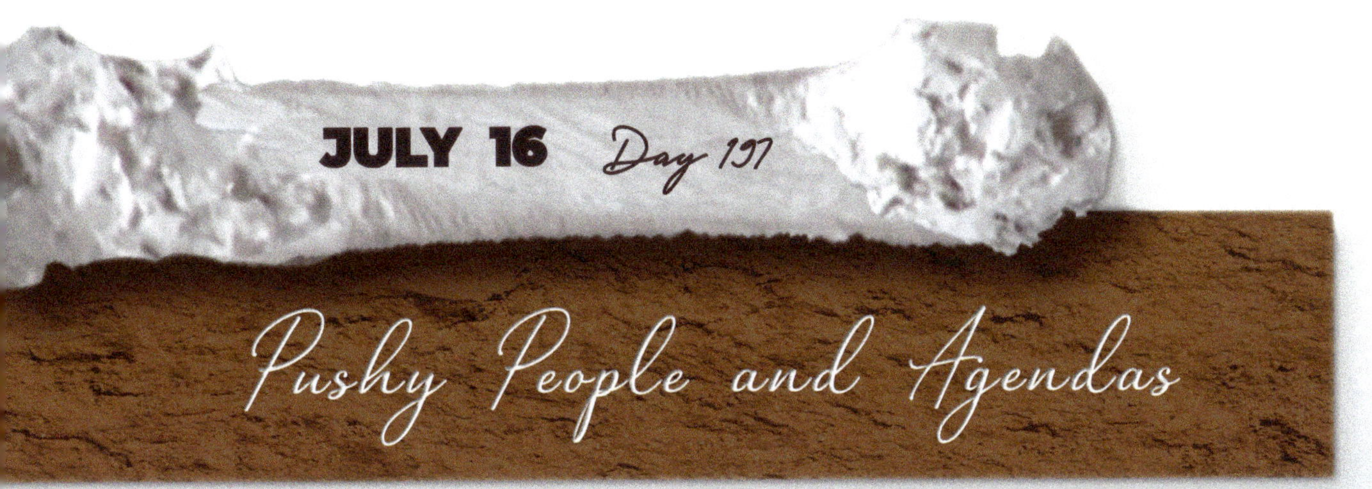

JULY 16 *Day 197*

Pushy People and Agendas

Coping with pushy people and agendas is unpleasant and challenging. One trick is trying to maneuver around them. However, avoiding someone is not always possible. It is more difficult to do when they are a friend or someone standing on your doorstep pretending they are doing you favors by selling you things. Learning how to read and recognize someone's agenda may be a simple tactic for boosting your time-management, effectiveness, assertiveness, and confidence in life. By reflecting a bit, you become more aware of pushy people, tactics, and their agendas.[209]

Today I will consider pushy people. Take it one step further and evaluate their agenda and how this may create stress for you. If it is your boss, perhaps try to think about their underlying work agenda. Everyone is subject to agendas. We are subject to the agendas of others and our own. Journal about a time you had to deal with a pushy person. What was the circumstance? Were you able to avoid that person, or did you overcome a situation? Are you good at reading agendas?

Courtesy of Umberto Kamperveen

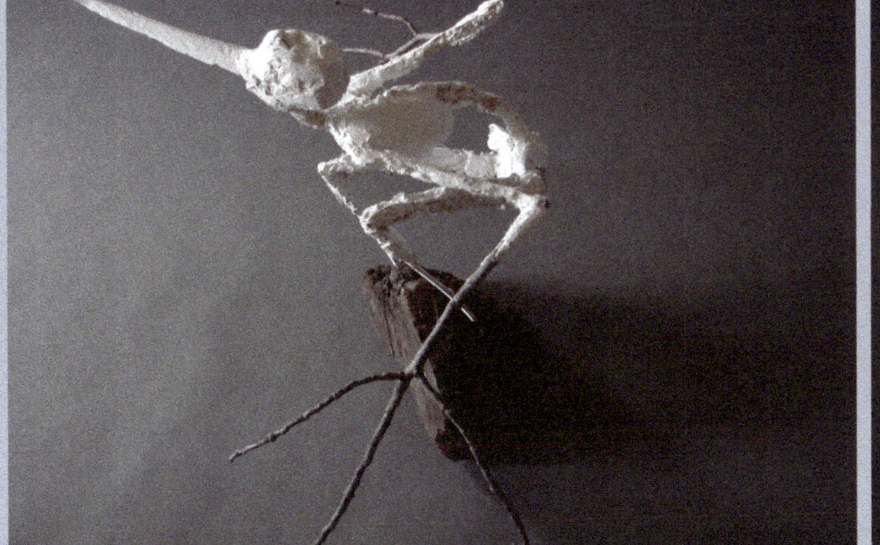

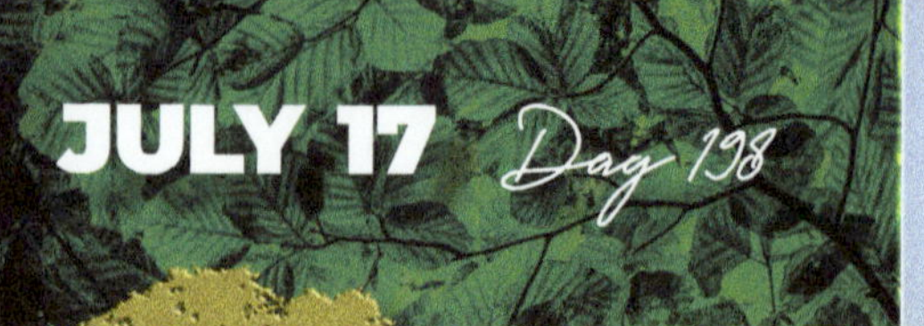

Elder Care and Working

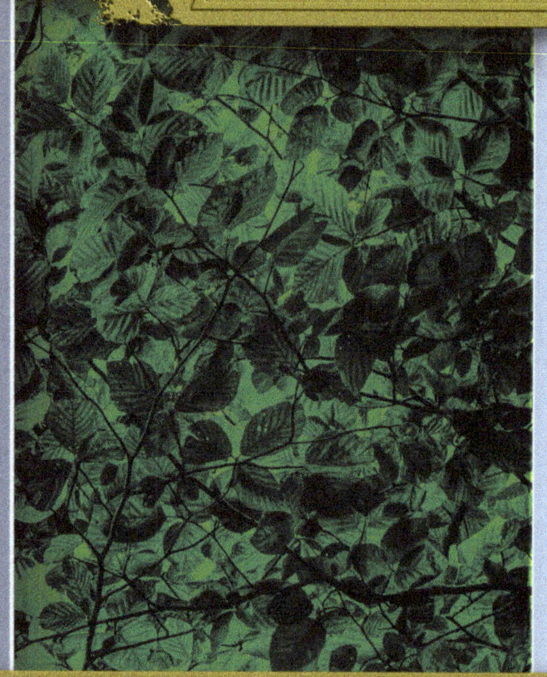

Current research has shown an increase in the number of caregivers handling dual roles. Not only are they working a full-time job, but also administering full-time care for an elder loved one. These types of caregivers are essentially working two full-time jobs. The way U.S. healthcare services are set up presently, family members are expected to provide immediate care for their elders with chronic illnesses, such as dementia. These expectations cause issues for family members, adult children, and spouses that must be effective at their jobs, be present and provide comprehensive care for an elder, and be available for their own family.[210]

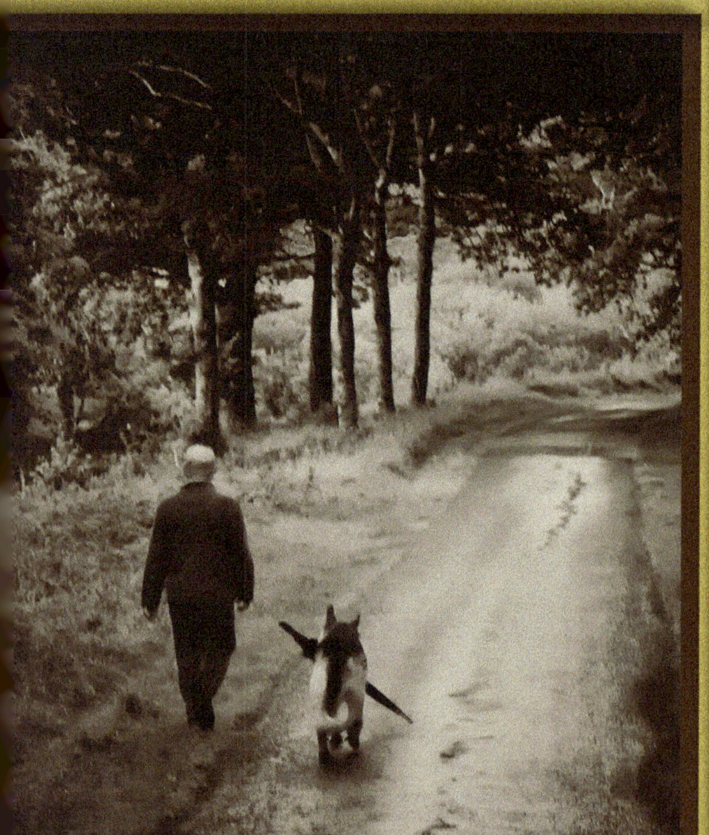

Today I will think about how I and many others may be caring for an elderly parent or relative and how that may create stress. They work their full-time job and then go home to another full-time job. Supporting others or finding the help you need to care for an elder and work full-time is essential in preventing burnout. Not everyone has access to the same resources. Let family and friends know that you need support. Ask for support. Journal about you or someone you know who is living a double-duty life. What does a typical day look like? How is it possible to balance all the responsibilities?

Courtesy of Rebecca Samler

Overcommitting

Always answering in the affirmative to invitations doesn't equate to kindness. It can take years to understand this concept. It doesn't always bring feelings of accomplishment. Knowing the difference between a true or obligated 'yes' can be a major breakthrough for a person. Take some quiet and reflective time to tell yourself the truth about your emotional state before answering. Commit to having relational limits and transparency. It's disingenuous to give so much time and energy away to be perceived as nice. Frankly, there are way too many helpful and pleasant individuals with undeveloped aspirations "dying on the vine." Overcommitting keeps us from what we really want. We do too much for others and are quick to dismiss our goals while rushing to assist others to achieve theirs. We neglect our aspirations because we overcommit, don't have energy, and this is a cycle.[211]

Today I will be aware of any "overcommitting" behaviors on my part. Recapture quiet time to reflect on your goals, projects, and dreams you want to accomplish. Journal about a time you overcommitted and how it felt. Did you feel any moral distress? Did you over-commit to things just to try and please others? How can you learn to say no and prevent over-committing in the future? It's okay to be a little selfish, especially when it comes to your personal time off and what is important to you.

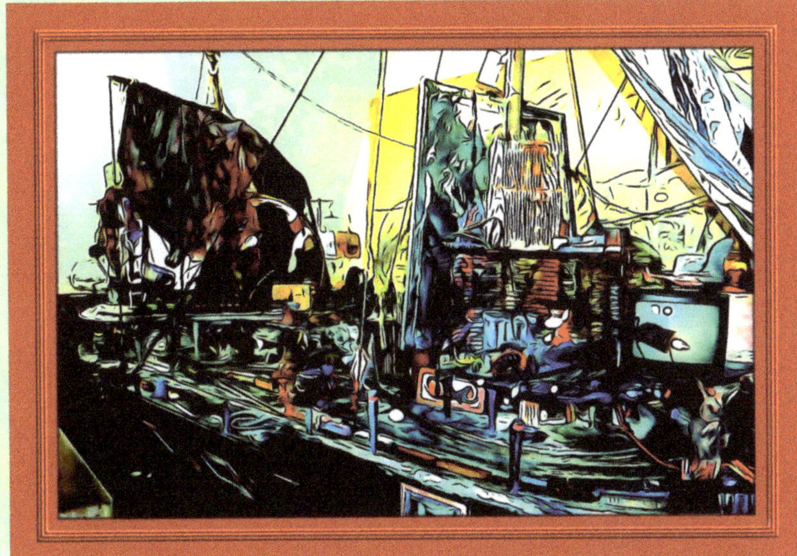

Courtesy of Robert John Holland

JULY 19

Day 200

Spending Time

It is important to nurture the special relationships of your life once they consist of the right people. Professionals agree that it is much easier to lose friends than make them. Stay connected with loved ones by offering encouragement, sympathy, and calling to check-in. Spend time not just when you want something – but also to let them know they are special to you. Be available for friends, and schedule time if needed.[212]

Courtesy of Linda Probst

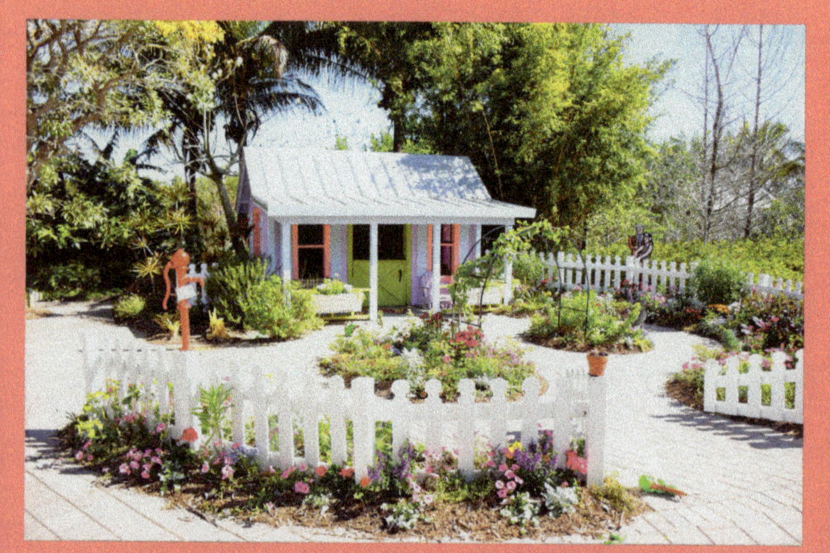

Today, after getting home from work, I will make an effort to spend time with family members or friends. Life isn't always about work; it's about enjoyment too. Your friends and family nurture your soul. They give you a sense of belonging in this world. Spending time with family and friends can often relieve stress, especially if they are supportive of you. Journal about the last time you made a family member or friend feel special, even if it was just a phone call. Do your family members or friends do the same for you? Do you tend to be better at making friends or losing them?

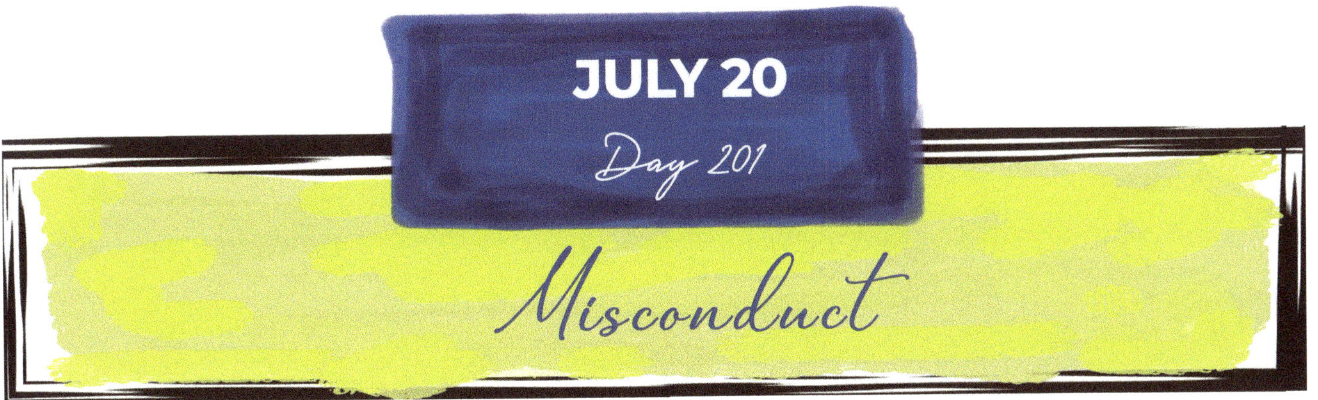

JULY 20

Day 201

Misconduct

Gross misconduct is related to severe employee behaviors. Determining whether a situation is genuinely blatant misconduct must not be restricted to the employer's inquiry. There is no single factor that is given more importance than another. The entire context must be taken into consideration when deciding on circumstances of misconduct. Certain actions or behaviors of an employee will usually add up to wrongdoing. There are many examples of blatant misconduct, including dishonesty, malicious damage, gross negligence, theft, breach of company policy, physical violence, fraud, and so on.[213]

Today I will consider my behavior and the actions of others at work. Journal about your workplace environment. Do you know of an instance where one of your coworkers was found to engage in misconduct, such as sexual harassment? This type of behavior creates stress and an unsafe atmosphere in the workplace. If these things occur regularly in your workplace, perhaps it is time to report it and/or find a new opportunity. You don't have to put up with this.

Courtesy of Edward Berkise

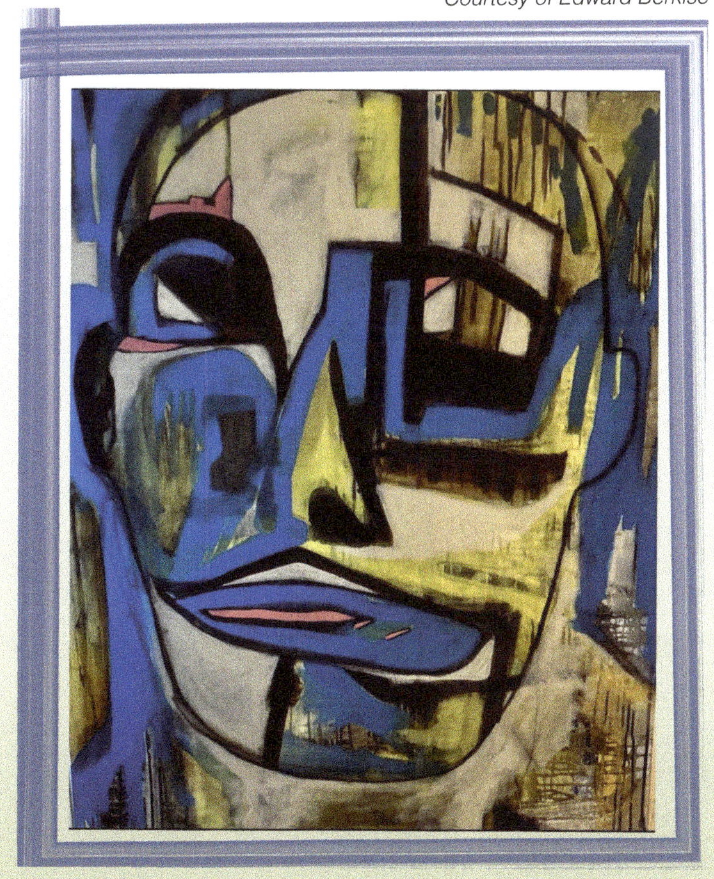

JULY 21

Day 202

Divisions

It is quite rare to enter offices today without finding noticeable divisions between groups of people within the room. Tight-knit coworkers share their lunch tables while they're on break discussing their latest projects. Or they buy each other rounds of drinks after the workday. Employees migrate between offices as they target employees who share the same opinions, work ethics, lifestyles, beliefs, career goals, as well as many other behaviors, mentalities, or emotions. Bonding in small groups allows them to dictate their workplace culture in productive, unique, and sometimes frightening ways. There are some negative environments and others that are highly professional. People can come together, mentor each other, collaborate, and even form a stronger company.[214]

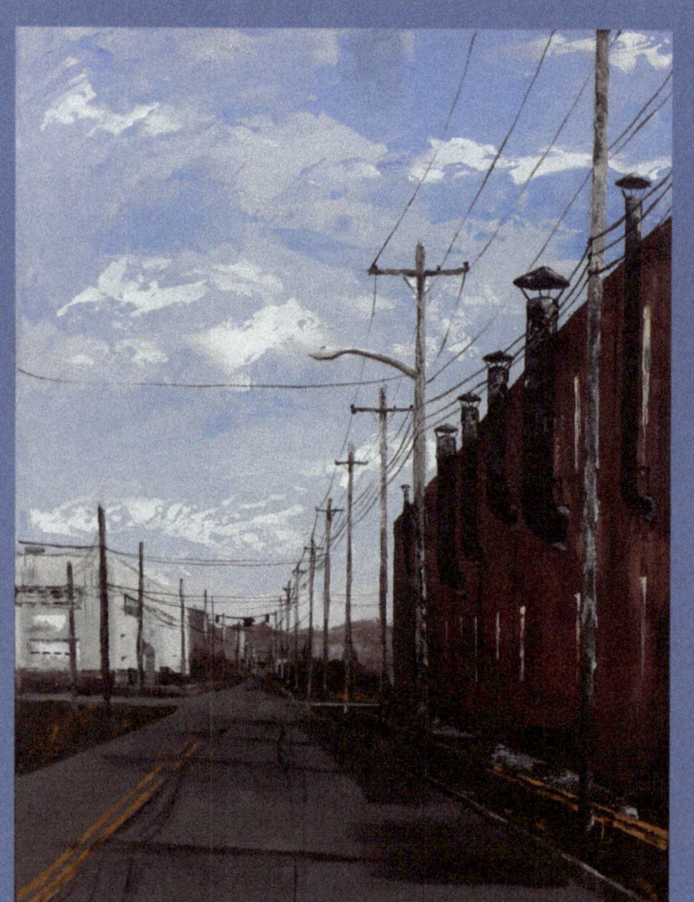

Today I will consider whether I am part of a small group at work. Reflect on the following in your journal. Is your group alienating another person or a newly hired coworker? Be mindful of how distancing from others may be harmful to those who are new. Tell yourself that you will make a conscious effort to be more inclusive of others, especially those that disagree with your opinions. What steps can you take to help bring unity to your workplace so everyone feels included?

Courtesy of Susan Gutierrez

JULY 22

Day 203

Being Relevant

An old lady would walk to a nearby river each day to collect water. She would bring two buckets with her, fill them, and walk back to her cozy little house. One bucket was sturdy and strong and could hold its water safely; however, the second bucket had a slight crack that would leak water as she walked home. When she arrived, typically, half of the water in the second bucket was gone. One afternoon, the cracked bucket, who didn't feel important or as relevant as the bucket without a leak, apologized to the lady. The cracked bucket said, "I'm terribly sorry for my defect. I will understand you replacing me with a perfect bucket." The old lady grinned. "Do you think I didn't know about that crack?" she asked. "Take a look at all the gorgeous flowers that happen to bloom and spread along the pathway from the river to home. I may have planted the seeds, but it was you each day doing the watering."[215]

Today I will think about my own "cracked bucket." Does the crack have to be a negative aspect, or can it be the very thing that makes you relevant? Consider the trail of flowers that grow from the leaking water in your cracked bucket. Use your journal to describe your imperfection and the relevance it may have in your life.

Courtesy of Spar Ki

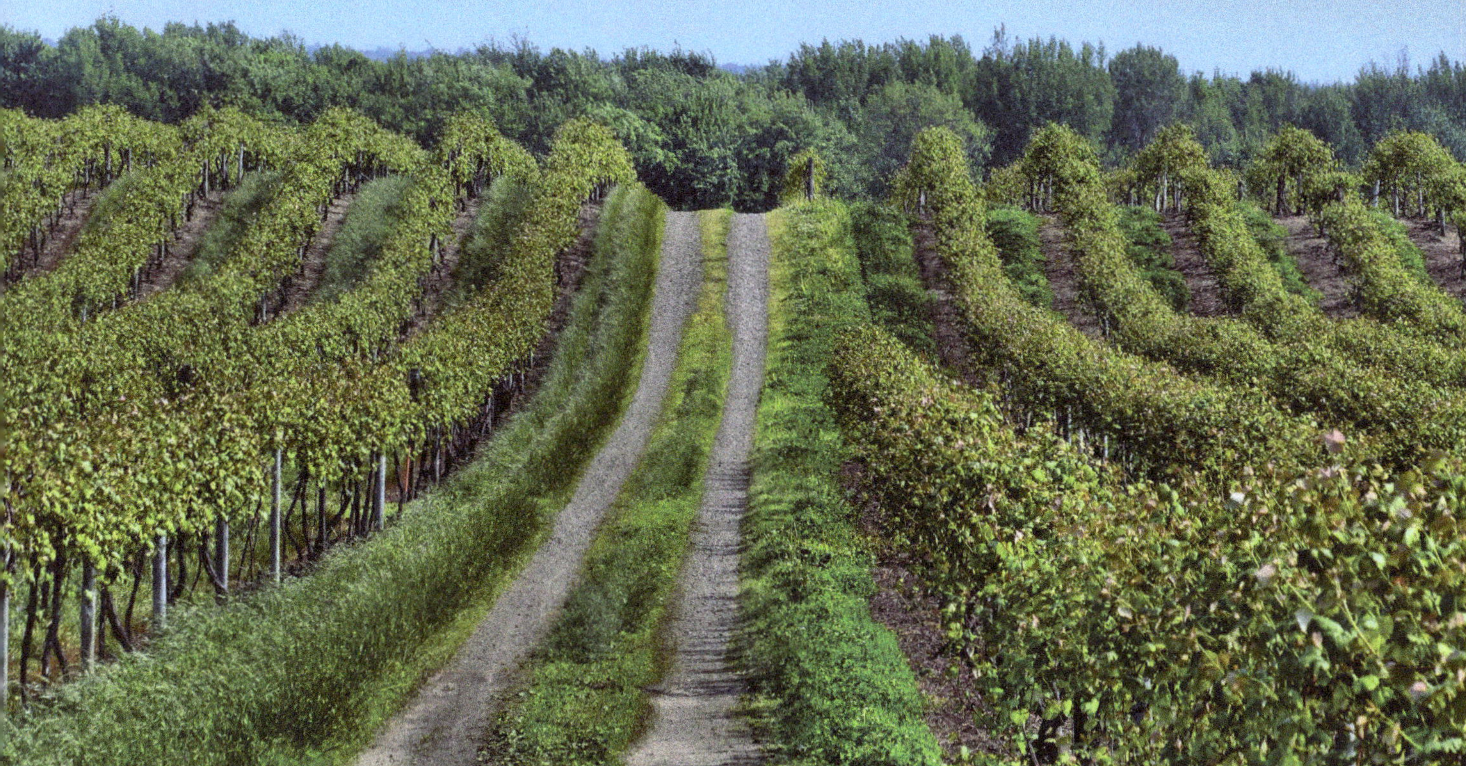

JULY 23

Day 204

Harmony

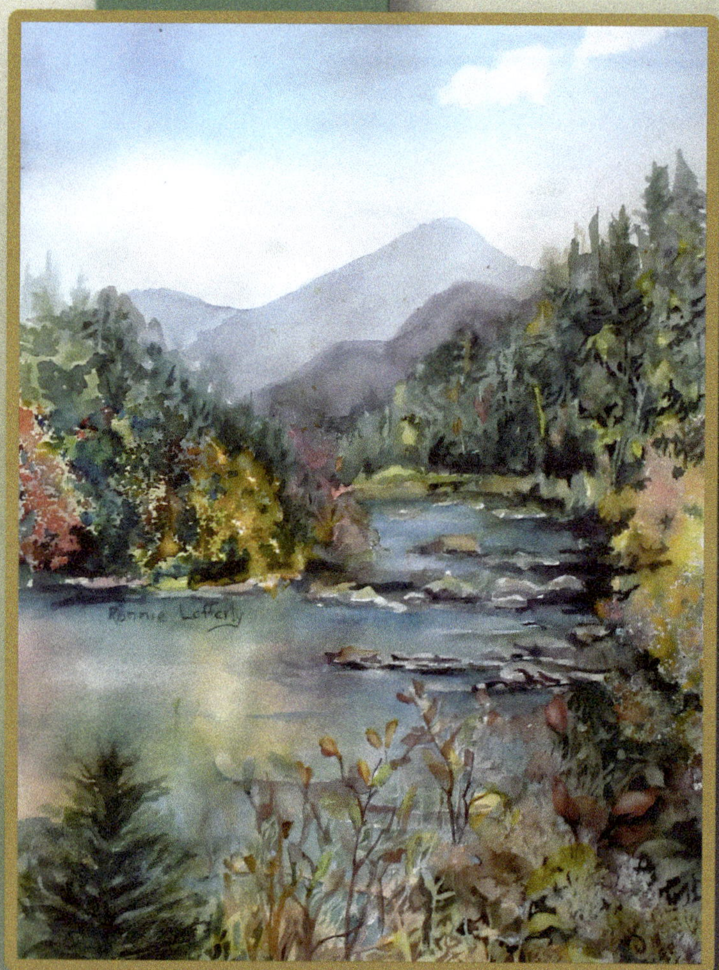

Courtesy of Ronnie Lafferty

"Offices are a microcosm of humanity." They include a mixture of many kinds of people with unique personalities, goals, challenges, and quirks. For each person to cooperate peacefully, it takes work. You've probably experienced a time in your career when a "clash of personalities" disrupted a constructive work environment. You can stop this from occurring and create harmony within your workspace.[216]

Today I will consider the things that I can do to create a more harmonious workplace. Creating harmony begins with me. Taking the time to build constructive relationships at work leads to peaceful environments. Journal about three things that you consciously do to create harmony at work and home.

Setting Boundaries

Setting healthy boundaries can do great things for a career. However, there's much more to the process than simply learning how to tell your boss no - although that is an important piece of the puzzle. You must also keep healthy and clear boundaries with coworkers, clients, and friends at work. Unfortunately, setting boundaries isn't exactly an easy thing to do. The tone you set with your professional relationships makes a large impact on your career. You must establish proper limits to help you become your best. It's crucial to set strict boundaries for those relationships to flourish. Also, it will assist you in feeling confident and relaxed. You will most likely end up enjoying your workday more.[217]

Today I will reflect on the boundaries I have set at work. Do you have boundaries? Can you identify what they are? Allowing others to interrupt while you are focused on what you are doing may cause a delay in your deadline. Is your deadline flexible? Is your teammates' need more urgent? Being able to say no when it is appropriate is okay when setting boundaries. Use your journal to answer.

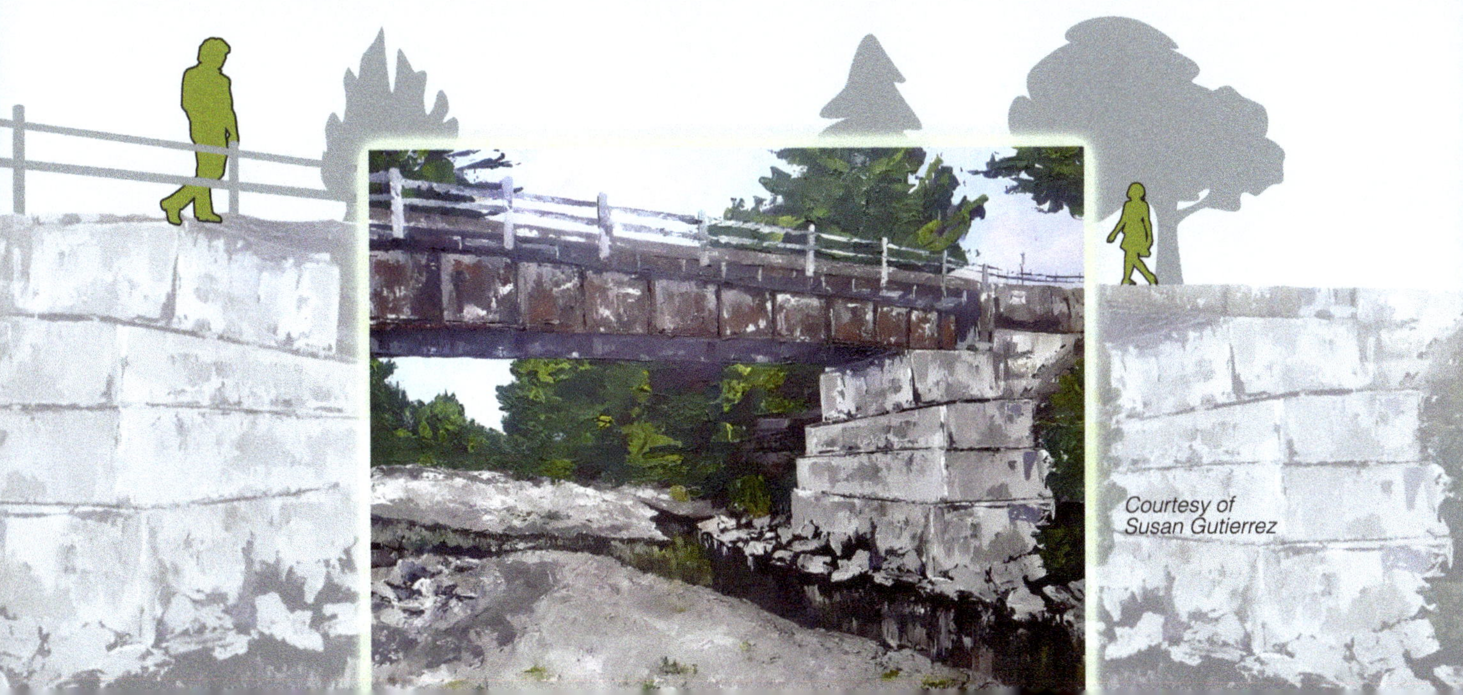

Courtesy of
Susan Gutierrez

JULY 25

Day 206

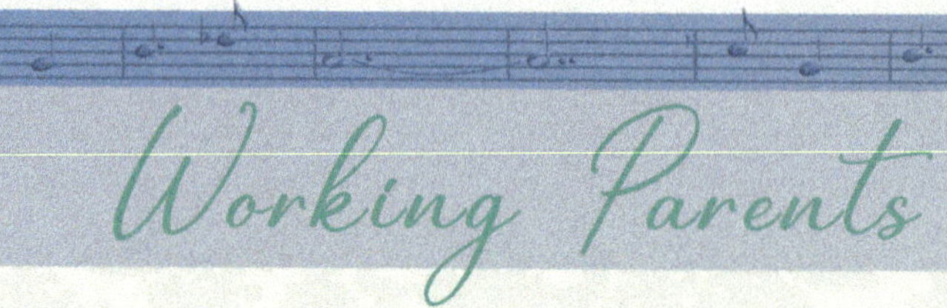

Working Parents

Childcare costs are not affordable, but not working is even more unaffordable. In either situation, a fiscal safety net may seem unachievable. You may be scared, angry, and questioning your choices. It's not surprising that parents choose hesitantly to quit working so they may be able to care for children. Of many industrialized countries, the U.S. doesn't offer paid leave for families. The country remains sadly underfunded when discussing childcare.[218]

Today I will be aware of the burden childcare costs are to Americans. When families are burdened with these costs, this creates panic and stress. When parents must remain home because of a chronically sick child, they often have to quit their jobs. Making it through the day, week, or month with so much stress on the family is remarkable. Journal about you or someone you know in the situation of working versus childcare. Is it possible to balance both? What would you say is the best solution once having children? Stay home, work full-time and hire help, or try and do both?

Courtesy of Toni Kelly

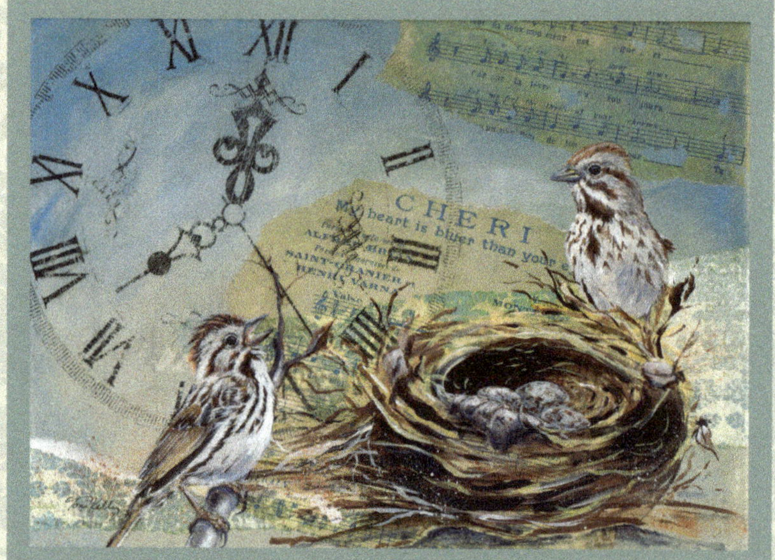

Generations at Work

When connecting employees with each generation, seven values matter most. These values are important to workers of any age. They include:

- Being listened to
- Feeling respected
- Having the opportunity for mentoring
- Being able to understand the bigger picture
- Receiving useful communication
- Having free idea exchange
- Obtaining positive feedback[219]

Today I will acknowledge that the variety of generations at work can be somewhat challenging and stressful. Different generations have different working styles and ethics. However, think about the common things each generation expects in the workplace. Respecting, listening, mentorship, shared vision, communicating well, and being evaluated fairly are some of the major things. Try doing these things when you are stressed or challenged in the moment. Journal about generation experiences you've encountered at work. What values are most important to you?

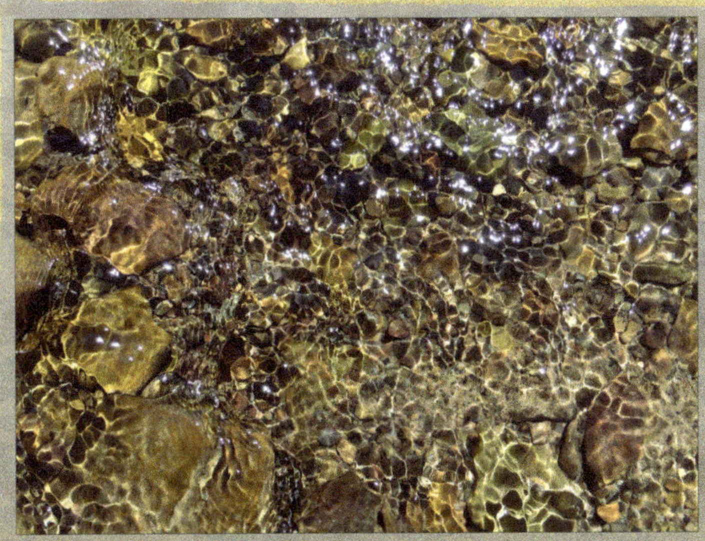

Courtesy of Barbara DelMonte

July 27

Taking a ME Day

Day 208

The busier our lives get, the quicker time appears to pass by. We tend to work ourselves to the max, spread ourselves thin, and direct attention less to our own needs. When we allow our career ambitions and everyday hustle to dominate our lives, we begin to feel exhausted. Working hard doesn't mean you don't like or appreciate your life as a partner, employee, or parent; however, losing yourself can rob you of your life passions and cause you to feel lost in your journeys. To avoid losing yourself, take some time off, and do things you enjoy. This is one of the best things for you and others around you.[220]

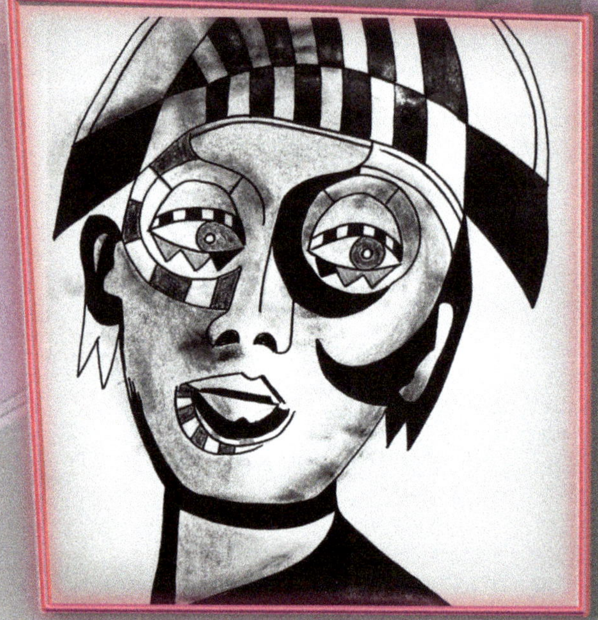

Courtesy of Edward Berkise

Today, I am going to plan a "ME" day. It's time for a drive in the country, brisk jog or walk in nature, yoga or martial arts, naptime, healthy meal, a small gift of something you have needed or wanted. Go ahead. Don't wait for someone to say you're worth it. Journal about your favorite "ME" time activities. What is your favorite way of alleviating stress and taking time for yourself?

JULY
28

Day 209

Meditation and Mindfulness

If you have been somewhat curious about meditation and mindfulness, make a commitment to a daily ritual. Begin with choosing a specific amount of time that is easily achievable – perhaps 2-10 minutes each day. After doing this for a week, reassess and decide whether you want to meditate more.[221]

Today I will think about slowing my mind down a bit and sitting for a few minutes to breathe. Rest one hand on your stomach and another on your forehead. Inhale on the count of three through your nose, exhale on the count of three through your mouth. Do this for 11 cycles. Notice the sensations in your body, the deep relaxation that you feel. Try to do this once a day, at any time. Journal by describing three things you feel once you've done this activity.

Courtesy of Barbara DelMonte

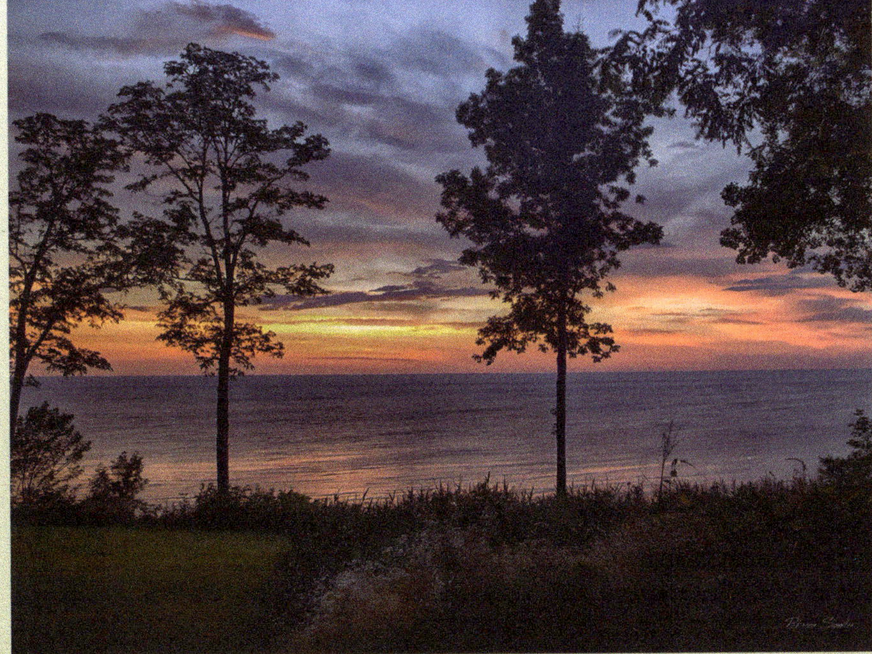

JULY 29

Day 210

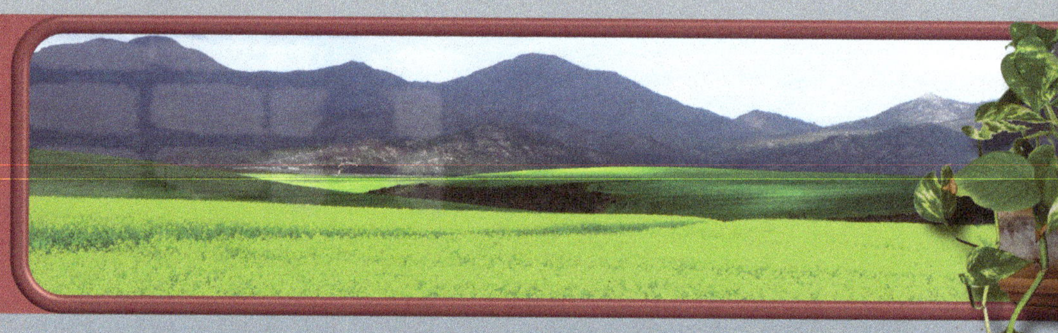

Looking Out the Window

Some may have more control over what they see outside of the window compared to others. Your ability to change your scenery by opening or closing your blinds is relevant. If you don't own a view with green nature outside, try adding some leafy green vegetation to the windowsill. When you see green, it boosts your performance and mood. You obtain bonus points when using various kinds of plants. Looking out the window at leafy green vegetation not only elicits a better mood and performance but is linked to a more creative mindset.[222]

Today I will look out my window. Do you like what you see? Your backdrop is important and can impact how you feel each day. If your view is not green, you can create a green space in your home. When you look out the window, what can you imagine, how far away can you see? Notice the relaxing sensation created by being still and looking out your window or at your green space. Write down everything you see and feel while looking out your window now.

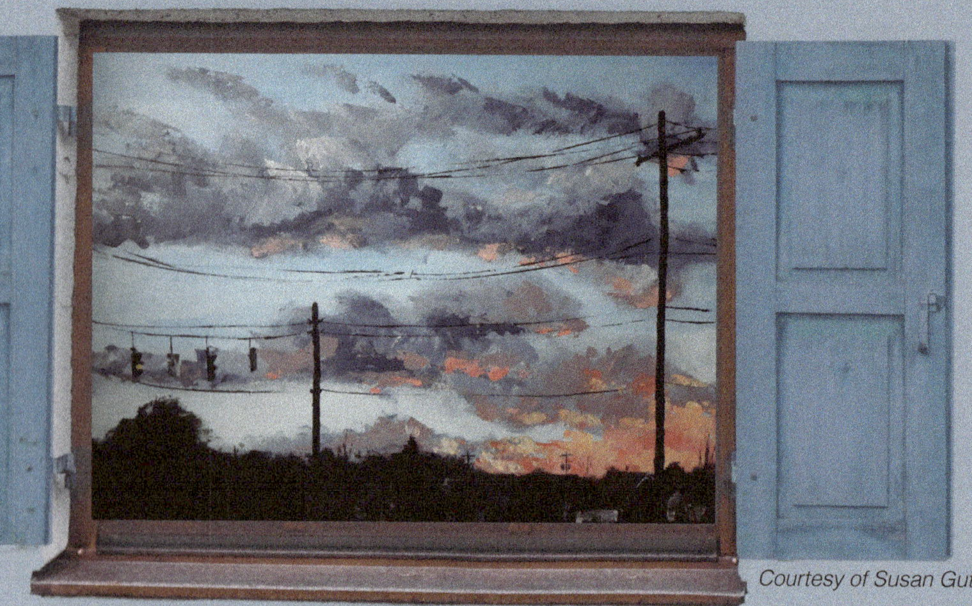

Courtesy of Susan Gutierrez

Personal Boundaries

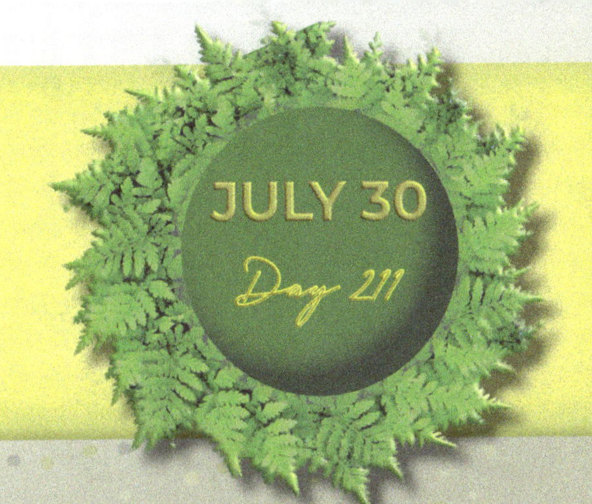

What is viewed as an appropriate boundary depends on the setting. Things that are appropriate to talk about with your friends might not be suitable in your workplace setting. Each culture has contrasting expectations when evaluating boundaries. For example, expressing emotions publicly can be considered highly inappropriate in some cultures, while other cultures encourage emotional expression.[223]

Today I will reflect on my personal boundaries. Setting boundaries is helpful because you know what to expect and what you can count on. Try to avoid overstepping boundaries and keep a healthy distance. Isolating oneself isn't always healthy but is sometimes physically necessary, and for introverts, it is normal. Know your boundaries, but don't forget to stretch them as well. Journal about what is important to you when it comes to personal space. Do you have different boundaries with your friends than coworkers? Are others aware of them?

Courtesy of Nancy Nixon Ensign

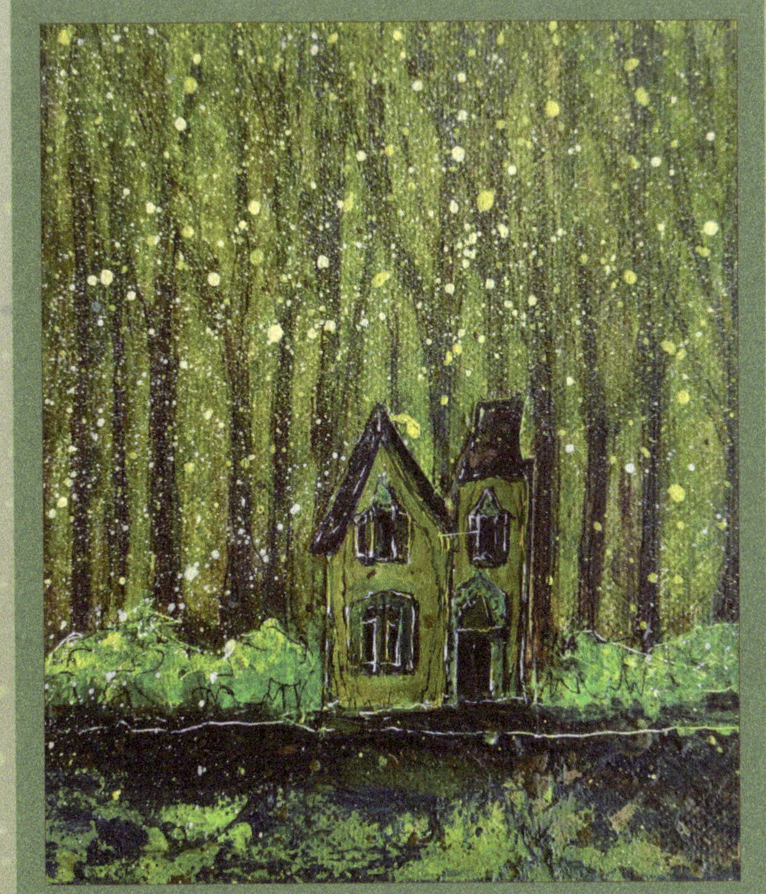

JULY 31

Day 212

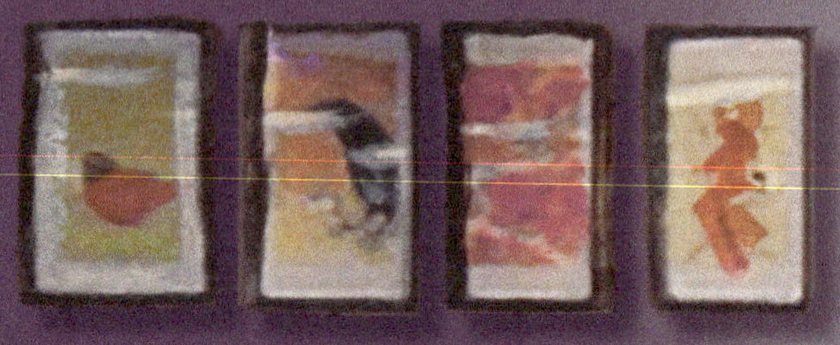

Avoid Gossip

Taking part in office gossip may seem tempting, but experts agree it might add stress while contributing to toxic work cultures. Thinking that listening to gossip is harmless if you keep quiet isn't true. It still changes your view of others in the workplace. You may have a tainted view of individuals or the organization you are working for by listening or engaging in gossip.[224]

Today I will notice who the gossipers are at work. Staying away from gossip is a conscious choice. Tell yourself that you are better than this and that you are not the type to participate. Gossiping is harmful to everyone and doesn't build esteem. Journal about gossiping that you have witnessed and the negative impact it had. What are ways you can avoid engaging in gossip? Do you try and discourage others from gossiping, or do you sometimes join in?

Courtesy of Susan MacKay

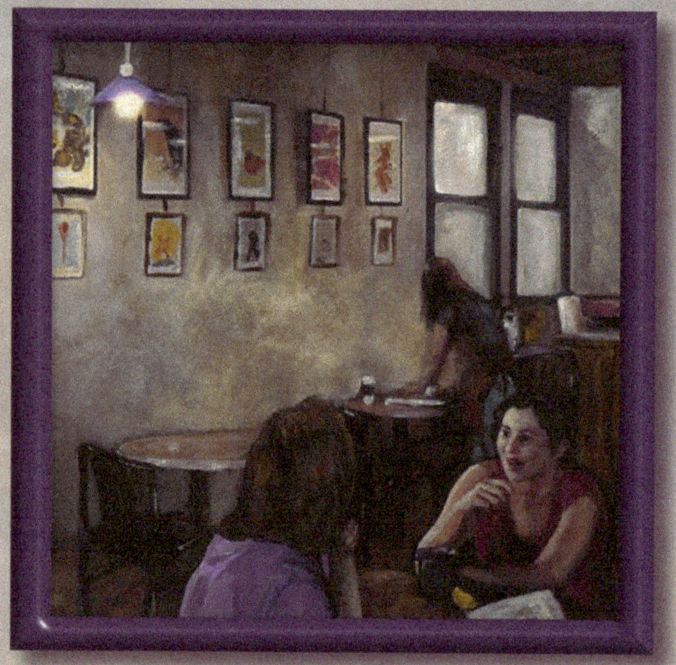

AUGUST 1

Day 213

Having PEP

"I can do prodigious work in an emergency, go without rest or eating when required because I have poise, efficiency, and peace."[225] -W. Hunter

Today I will calculate my poise, efficiency, and peace (PEP) level. Rate yourself from 1 at the lowest PEP to 10 at the highest. What number are you at? Sometimes you need a pulse check. Think about your poise, efficiency, and peace. Journal about a situation or example of how you exhibited each trait within the past week.

Courtesy of Eduardo Andres

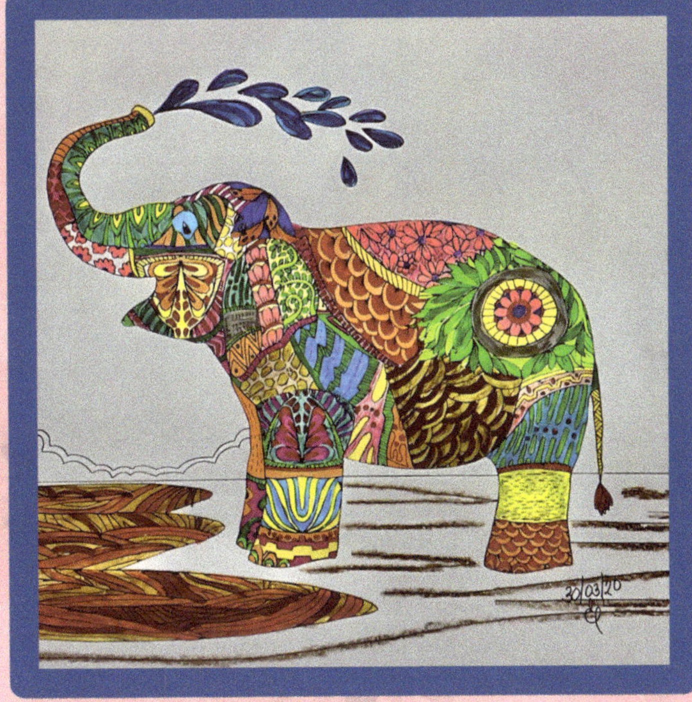

AUGUST 2

Day 214

Doubting Yourself

Self-doubt can destroy your heart, body, mind, and soul. Self-doubt is a major obstacle to living an authentic life and one that is truly deserved. Self-doubt is unhealthy food, harming your soul and dragging your spirit down. It crushes ambitions and blocks you from obtaining your goals and dreams.[226]

Courtesy of Umberto Kamperveen

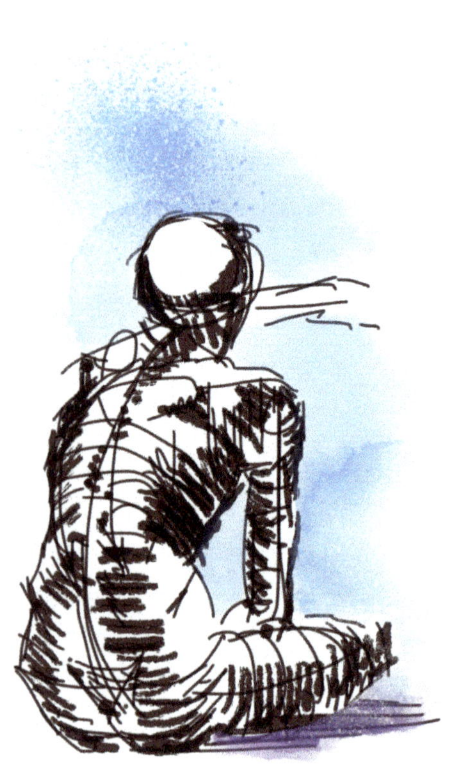

Today I will think about the last time I doubted myself. What was it about? Was it confidence related? Confidence and self-doubt seem to oppose each other. As your confidence level rises, your self-doubt decreases. Pay attention to inverse relationships. Write about what lifts your spirit, what drives your ambitions, and describe your last achievement in your journal.

AUGUST 3

Day 215

Grit

Grit can be described as having the passion and perseverance to reach your long-term goals. You may also hear grit defined as mental toughness.[227]

Today I will recollect some long-term goals I have obtained. For instance, finishing school, obtaining a satisfying job, creating a family, building wealth, or earning something of value. Reflect on what it took to reach those goals. That is what grit is - what it takes to achieve things. It's never too late to make a new goal and demonstrate grit. Journal about a time that you needed grit to accomplish something.

Courtesy of Spar Ki

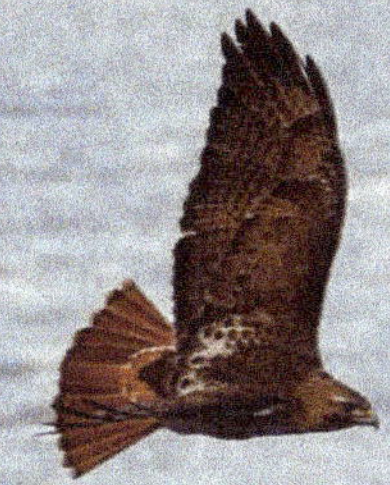

Privacy

The HOUPE study of university hospital physicians in four European countries considered client confidentiality and its role as a barrier for physicians seeking social support. The results indicated that client confidentiality is often linked to high role conflict, less control over the work pace, and less decision making, which creates emotional distress among physicians. Concerns to protect client privacy may be a drawback for obtaining and utilizing the social support of other physicians. Social support may change or lower emotional distress while patient confidentiality can increase distress by interrupting useful coping and adaptation methods.[228]

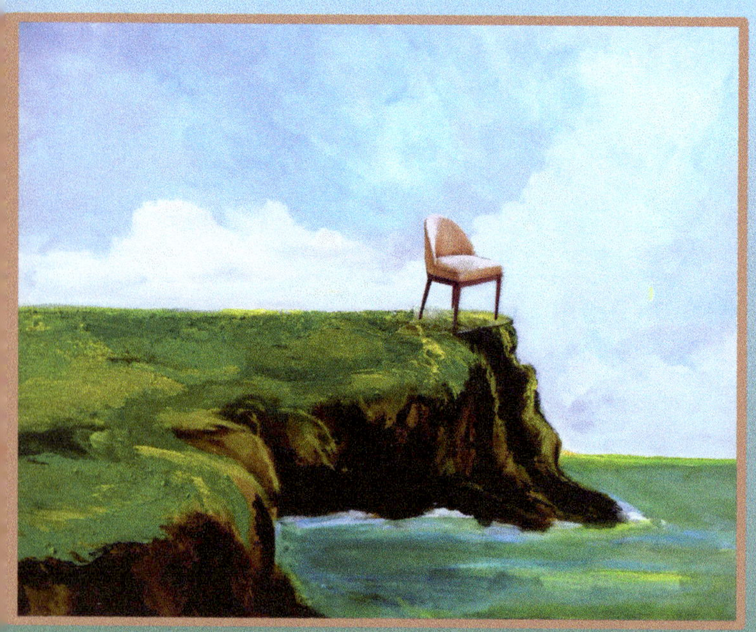

Courtesy of Nancy Nixon Ensign

Today I will consider how patient privacy may contribute to my stress and burnout. In your journal, can you write about a time when a client's privacy created a stressful situation? What happened? Did HIPAA (client privacy) cause an increase in workload, "red-tape," inability to debrief, or share information with other providers? How did you manage the privacy concern?

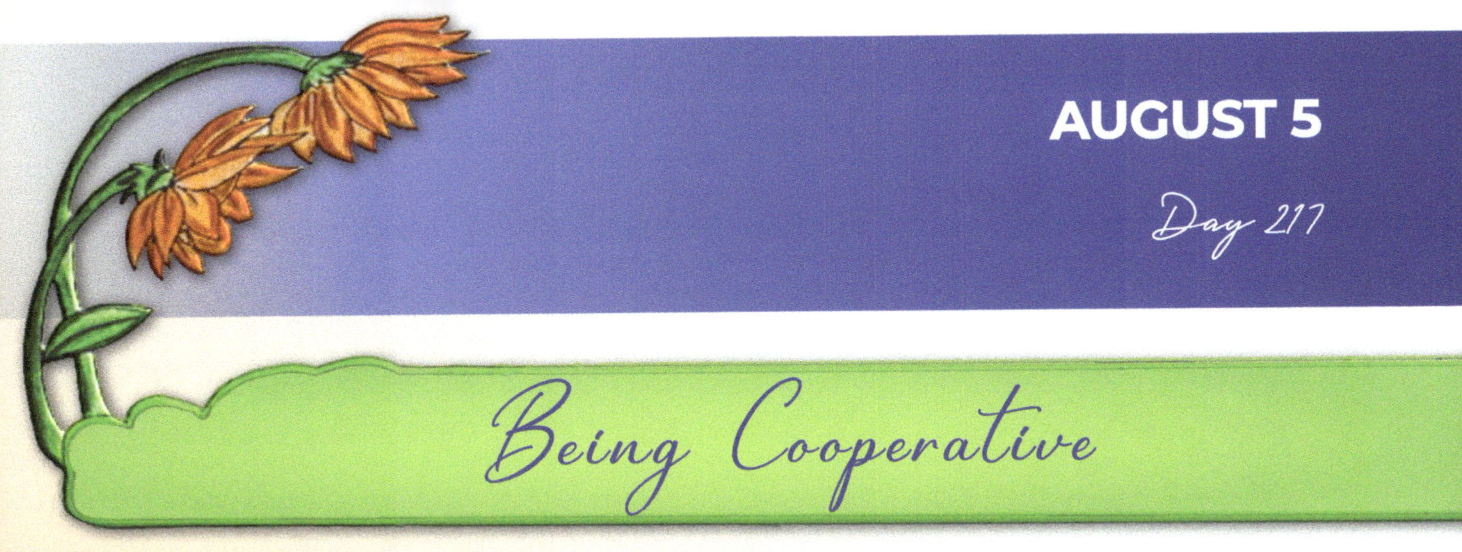

AUGUST 5

Day 217

Being Cooperative

Are you someone who purposefully and frequently helps coworkers with strenuous tasks or crucial presentations? You may think it can strengthen your reputation and increase your popularity, but science proves that excessive professional kindness may have the opposite effect. Highly generous and cooperative people tend to attract more social punishment and hatred than deserved. This is especially clear in competitive environments, such as a populous workplace. People seem inclined to treat those who behave overly friendly with suspicion and hostility. This is reminiscent of similar behaviors displayed with ancient humans in hunter-gathering groups.[229]

Today I will consider how being overly cooperative may attract unkind treatment. Journal about a time at work when you were overly kind, and it didn't really create the effect you intended or even backfired. Has this ever happened to you? How competitive is your work environment? Do you have a suspicion about overly cooperative people? Are you overly cooperative?

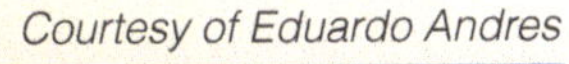

Courtesy of Eduardo Andres

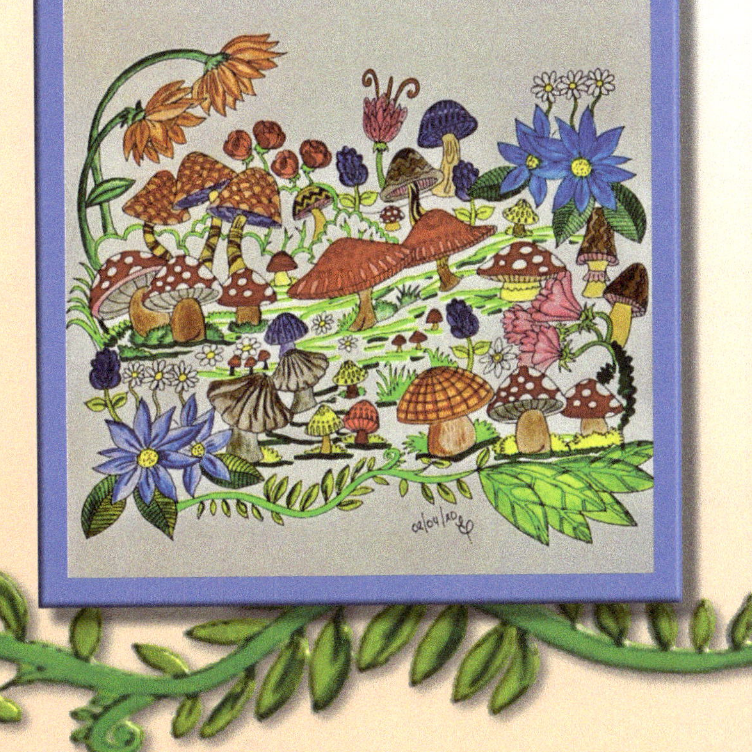

Setting New SMART Goals

- SMART goals are Specific, well-defined, unambiguous, and clear.
- SMART goals are Measurable and contain specific criteria, measuring progress towards goal accomplishment.
- SMART goals are Achievable and attainable, not impossible.
- SMART goals are Realistic, reachable, and relevant.
- SMART goals are Timely and create urgency. They have defined timelines with a start date and target date.[230]

Today I will think about a new SMART goal that I want to set, related to my career or some sort of progress that I want to make. Journal about your new SMART goal and the timeline you need to achieve success.

Courtesy of Toni Kelly

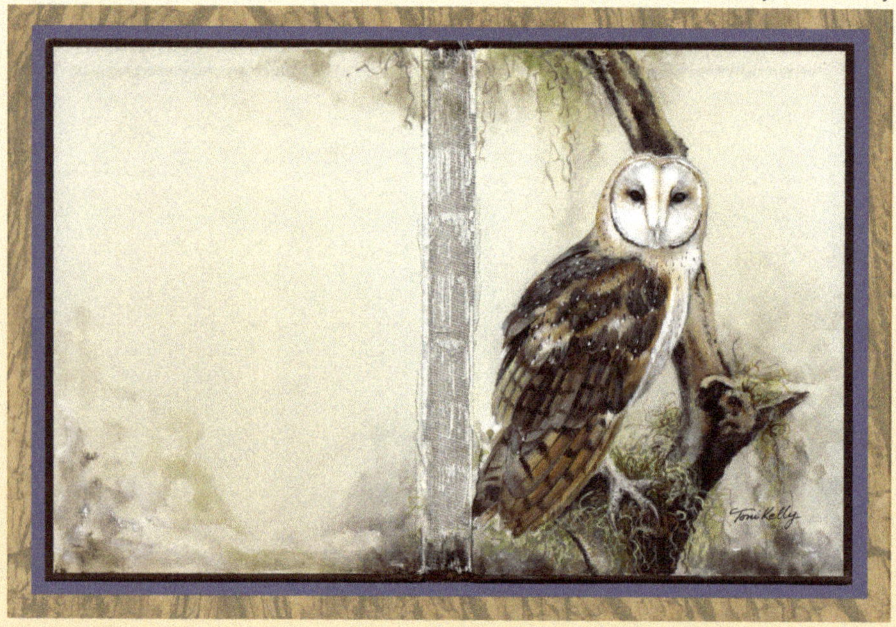

AUGUST 7

Day 219

Civility

It is an era of expanding political separations within the U.S., with many people divided on opposing political views. People are not only in disagreement; many are bordering on hate for the opposite side. This dislike has been increasing for decades. An NPR/PBS NewsHour/ Marist poll shows there is a growing lack of civility, and Americans are seeing violent disturbances and protests at government buildings, including the Capitol as a result. What meaning does civility truly have? At times, it is defined as being polite. It originates from the Latin root "civilis," which means "befitting a citizen." It is a term that puts some at ease and is uncomfortable for others. So "civility" includes politeness, but it consists of much more.[231]

Today consider civility at home, work, and in the community. The political divide has created so much stress in recent years, and it has undoubtedly caused weariness. The media compounds the incivility with news that may or may not be true. Journal about what you can do to create civility and describe two civil acts you have made within the past month that demonstrate peace and tolerance.

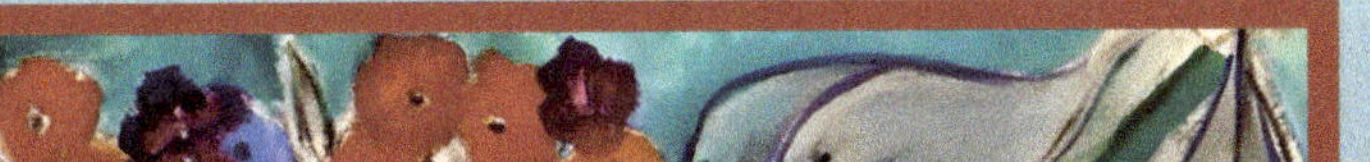

Courtesy of Maika Gonzalez

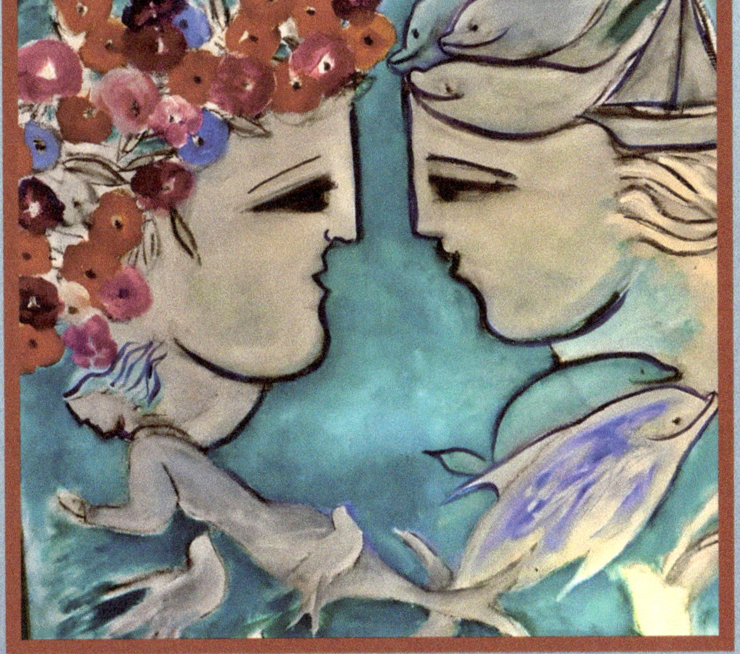

AUGUST 8

Day 220

Social Justice

The formal definitions of social justice vary. Certain commonalities exist. They include equality of rights, opportunities, and treatment. Having values such as these in mind can help us define the following phrase: ***"Social justice means equal rights, opportunity, and treatment for all."*** [232]

Today I will consider "social justice" and what it means to me and others. Poverty, race, and religion may create unfair treatment. Journal about how rights, opportunities, and treatment have affected you or someone you know. What things can you do to help others that may not have access to the same rights, opportunities, and treatment as you? List three ideas.

Courtesy of Jill Mattson

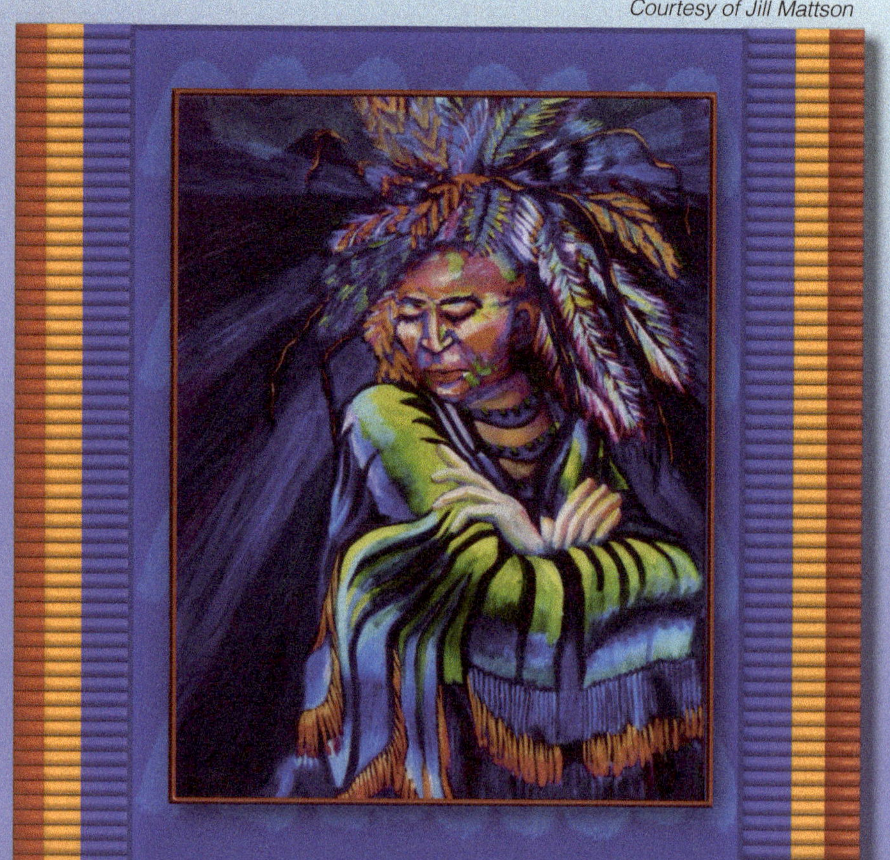

AUGUST 9

Day 221

Growing from Mistakes

Success isn't a fantasy or pot of gold at the end of a rainbow. Failure isn't always in terms of black or white. Life truly is ten percent what happens and ninety percent how we respond. Failure may be inspirational. It may just lead to bigger, better things. The only way we reach success is if we learn from failures and continue growing from mistakes.[233]

Today I will reflect on one mistake that I have made. Journal about whether you took accountability for it. In retrospect, write about what you also learned from your mistake and if you are better or worse off now. Do you feel that you have grown to be more successful after learning from your mistakes? Making mistakes can be stressful. Not owning up to mistakes can be a huge source of stress and burnout.

Courtesy of Barbara DelMonte

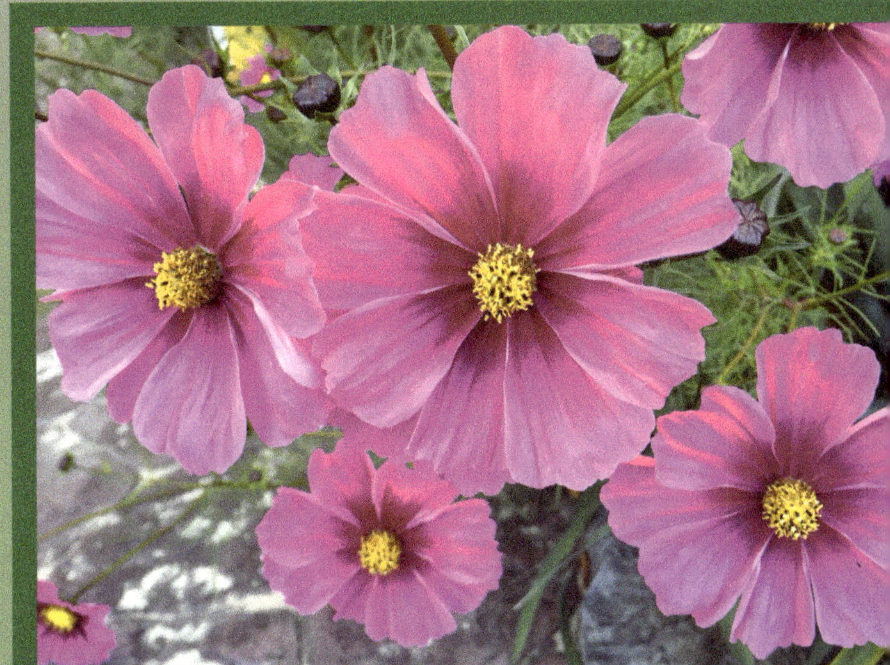

AUGUST 10

Day 222

Verbal Abuse at Work

The abuser isn't always the issue; it's the effect the abuser has on you. You can term it as bullying, psychological torture, emotional abuse, or verbal abuse. You name it to acknowledge it is hurting your performance at work and has emotional consequences. Next time an abuser disturbs you, stop them and inform them that what they are saying and doing is upsetting. Tell them that continuing that behavior will force you to report the issue to a manager. It may also be helpful to start searching for a new job. There is a chance that your boss won't be able to fully assist you in removing the abuser without just cause and proof. Your sanity and health are more valuable than your job, and verbal abuse at work tends to erode both.[234]

Today I will tell myself I do not have to take verbal abuse. You don't have to put up with it. Address it on the spot by telling the abuser you will report the behavior to management, escalating when necessary. Or you can make an alternative plan. The Joint Commission offers a Code of Conduct that can be found online as a resource for all team members to guide behaviors in the workplace. Use this time now to journal about your plan. Create a new vision for yourself and your career. Your sanity and health are at stake.

Courtesy of Robert John Holland

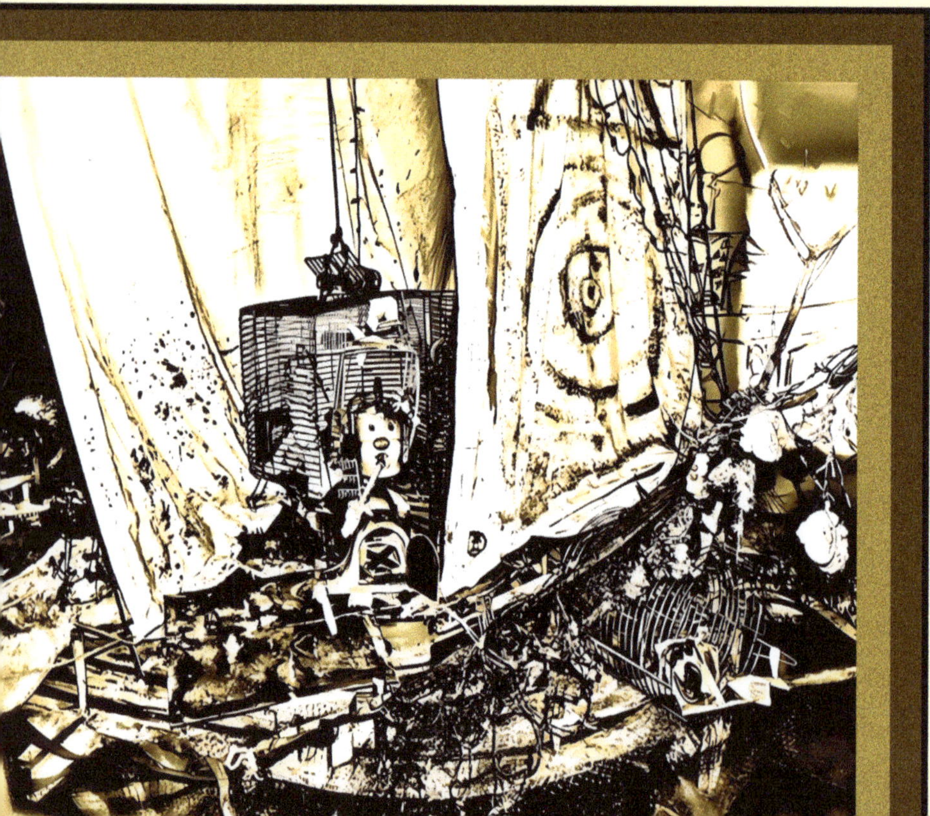

Making a Wish

When wishes come true, it produces transformation, hope, and strength. Making a wish has proven emotional and physical rewards that give critically ill children higher chances of surviving.[235]

Today I will make a wish for myself. Think about it for a few minutes. What wish do you want to come true? Can you see in your mind's eye what might happen? Imagine that. Use your senses: smelling, touching, hearing, seeing, tasting ... Journal about the wish you want to come true and manifest it. Set a timetable for it to happen. Is this a form of "magical thinking,"[236] and will it improve your chances of survival?

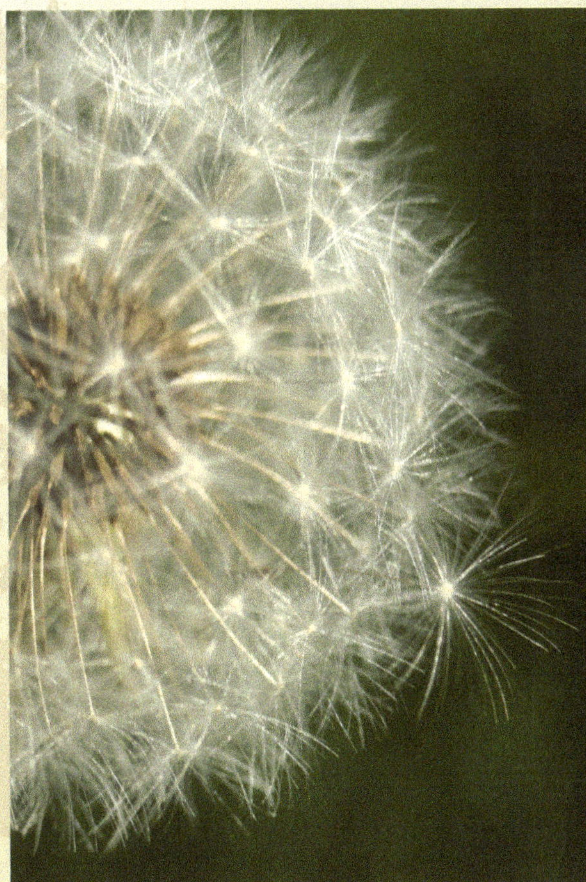

Courtesy of Barbara DelMonte

AUGUST 12

Day 224

Terminated

Being terminated is both a terrifying and humiliating experience. Despite the reasoning behind why you were terminated, you may feel as though you failed both the company and yourself. The scary part is fearing that you will never obtain another job. Many people get fired, and their ability to find another job is not affected. Employers often look more positively on the people who were terminated as opposed to those who quit without having another job lined up.[237]

Today I will reflect on whether I have been fired. Was it really your fault? There are many irrational, hostile, and arbitrary owners, managers, human resource professionals, and supervisors out there.[238] Journal about your experience or a friend's experience of being terminated. Are you or your friend better off now, or worse off? What did you learn from the experience? Describe your resilience.

Courtesy of Spar Ki

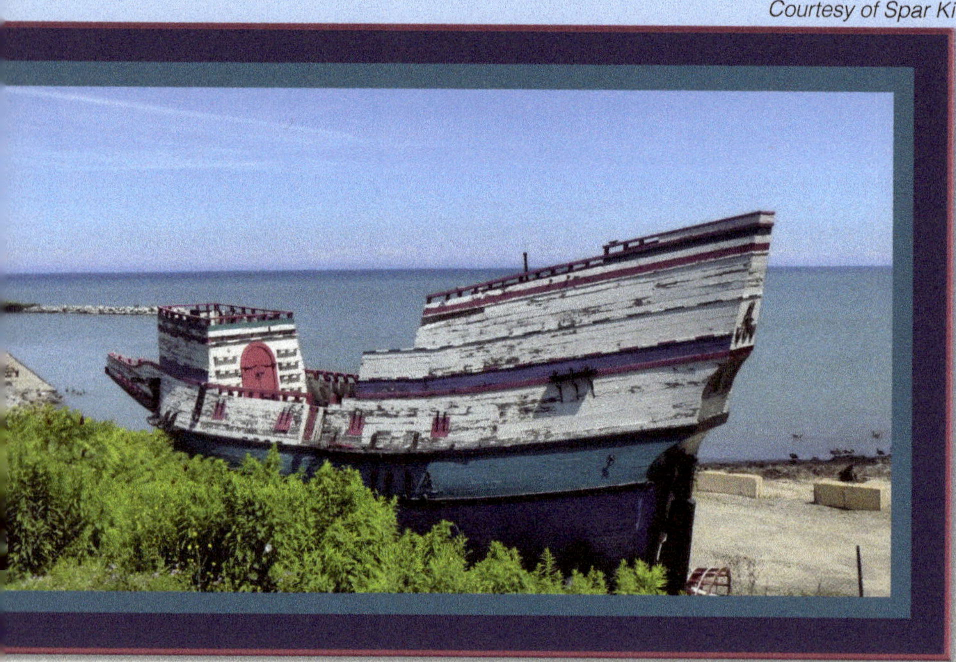

Having Your Back

Not everyone is your friend. Simply because you are spending time together, laughing, doesn't mean they're on your side. Having your back is more than just saying it. It means not stabbing you in the back. People easily pretend. Jealousy can be nearby. It's wise knowing your circle and paying attention because fake people can often be exposed in real situations.[239]

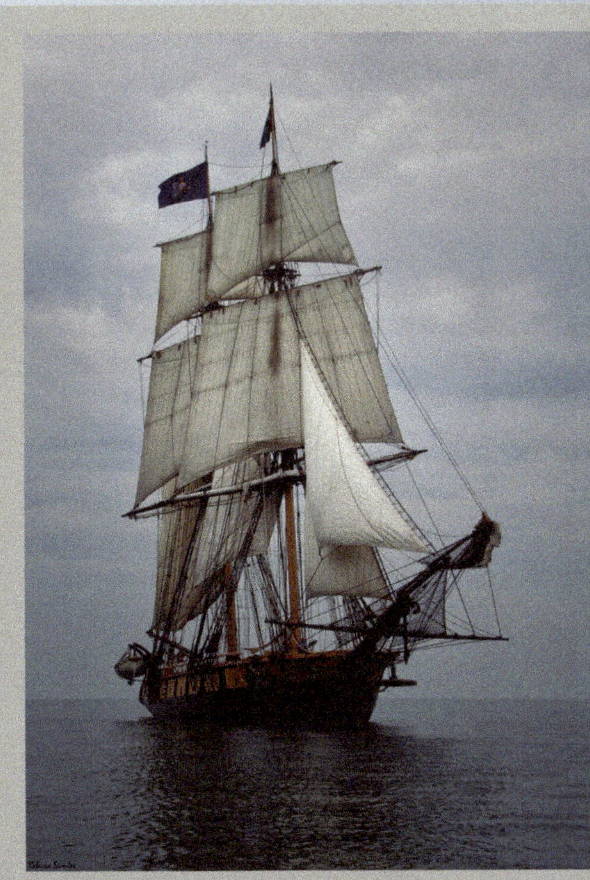
Courtesy of Rebecca Samler

Today consider who really has your back and who doesn't. Can you tell (most of the time) who the wolves are in sheep's clothing? Journal about a time when you thought someone had your back, but they didn't. Think about the stress, exhaustion, and disappointment this may have caused you. Do you connect how events like this can really lead to stress? Do you have others' backs?

AUGUST 14

Day 226

Concentrating on the Positive

Self-talk that is negative can creep up and be difficult to notice. It's easy to think that you are bad at something or should have never tried doing it. Negative thoughts become feelings that you internalize and may turn into concrete self-beliefs. Recognize when you are doing this and stop negative thoughts by concentrating on the positive. Then, replace those negative thoughts. Replace "I am no good at this" with "I will get more practice and improve." Thinking "I should have never tried" becomes "That did not work out so well; there's always next time."[240]

Today and each day, I will use positive thinking whenever I notice my negative thinking. Concentrating on this takes active self-awareness. Describe in your journal how you could have chosen to listen to negative self-talk, but you chose positive self-talk instead. What was the event going on? Were you able to continue concentrating on the positive thoughts days later? Be honest with yourself.

Courtesy of Jill Mattson

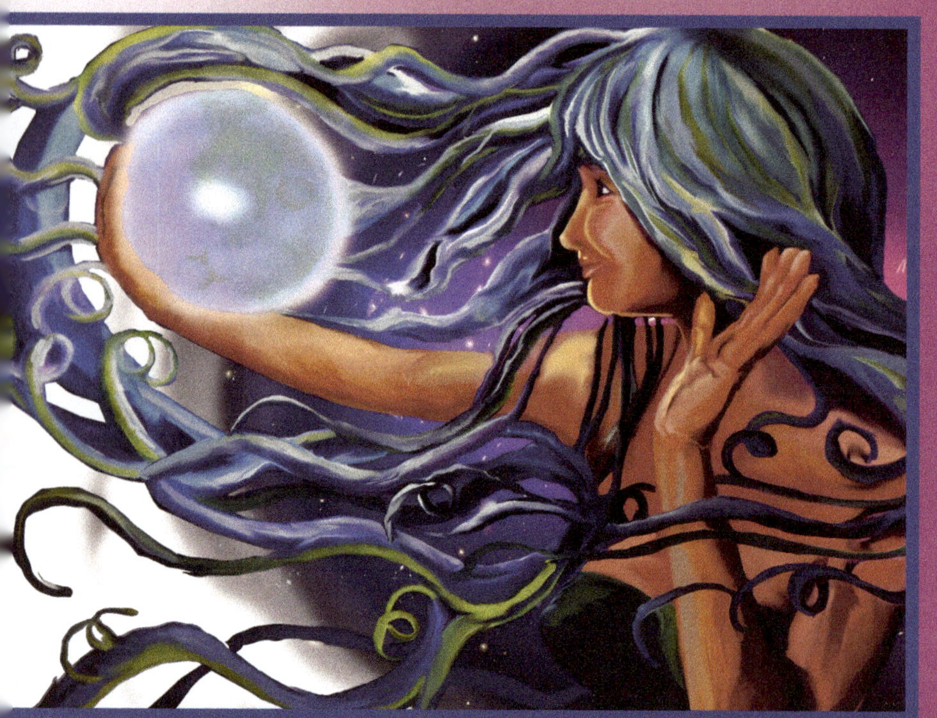

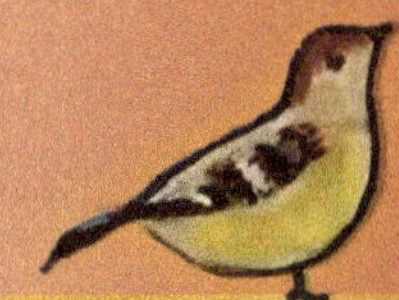

AUGUST 15

Day 227

Popularity

Unfortunately, the struggles of climbing social ladders did not finish after high school. "Desk eaters," or those who try sneaking into the office without saying hello to coworkers, will stay on the bottom of the ladder, both professionally and personally. Those who genuinely try climbing are the ones that achieve popularity. In fact, workplace popularity is associated with higher productivity, better treatment by teammates, greater visibility, as well as an increased likelihood of promotions or rewards.[241]

Today I will consider popularity and how unfortunate it is that career advancement is mostly based on it. It doesn't matter that you struggled your entire life to achieve and go to school collecting degrees and credentials. When it comes to advancing your career, those are the minimum qualifications in a competitive market. Sadly, it is about networking, who you know, and your popularity. If you are an introvert, it could be much more difficult to advance. Journal about how popularity has helped or hindered your career advancement. Think about how popularity can add to stress and burnout, especially if you are an introvert stuck in an extroverted hiring market.

Courtesy of Maika Gonzalez

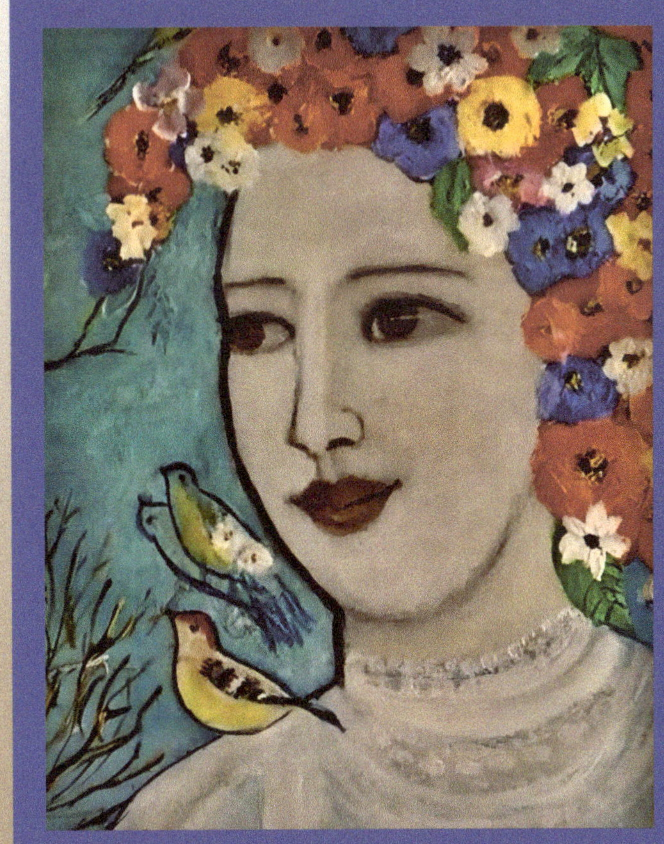

AUGUST 16

Day 228

Drawing the Line

Is there a "best friend" at work who you trust with information and fully share everything, from personal problems to workplace rants? Imagine discovering that this "friend" of yours ends up being the informant to someone in upper management. Everything you told them in confidence, whether it was innocent or not, had been conveyed to the boardroom throughout the years. This unfortunate circumstance is consequential when not drawing the line or keeping emotional boundaries at work. This is a most unfortunate lesson.[242]

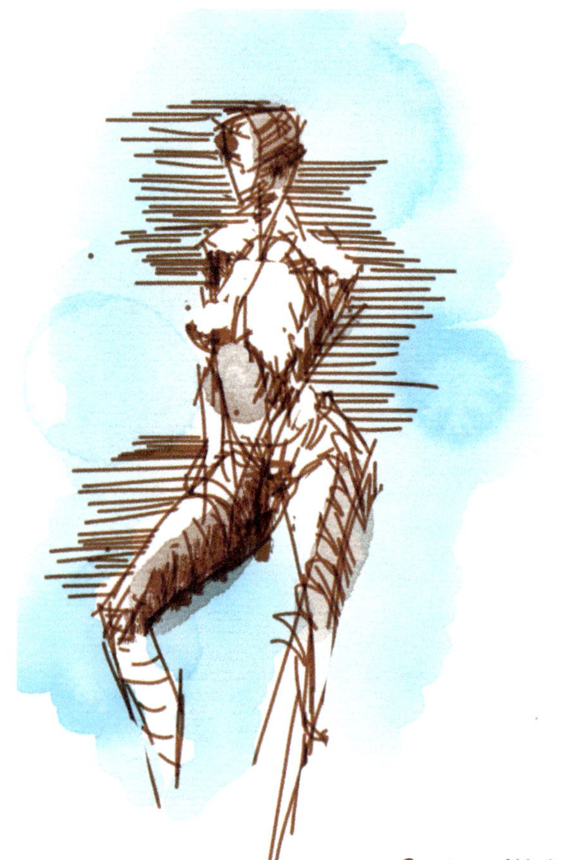

Courtesy of Umberto Kamperveen

Today I will consider that my "friend" at work may not really be my friend. Consider that sometimes "friends" are in reality "acquaintances" or "co-workers." This is a harsh reality in today's work climate, where trust and boundaries are challenged. Journal about a time that you told something to someone at work, and it got back to another person or your boss. Write about the stress this caused. Drawing the line by keeping safe boundaries is imperative to avoid being derailed.

Being Nimble

The world is hectic and evolving, and the pace is rapidly changing more than before. Therefore, it is crucial to be nimble and have the ability to adapt, react, "think on your feet," and be effective, quick, and positive.[243]

Today I will consider how nimble I am. You must be able to be quick to comprehend and seize the moment. Journal about a time you used your agility to capture one of your successes. Describe that success. What was the situation? Did you "think on your feet?" Are you quick to react and adapt?

Courtesy of Linda Probst

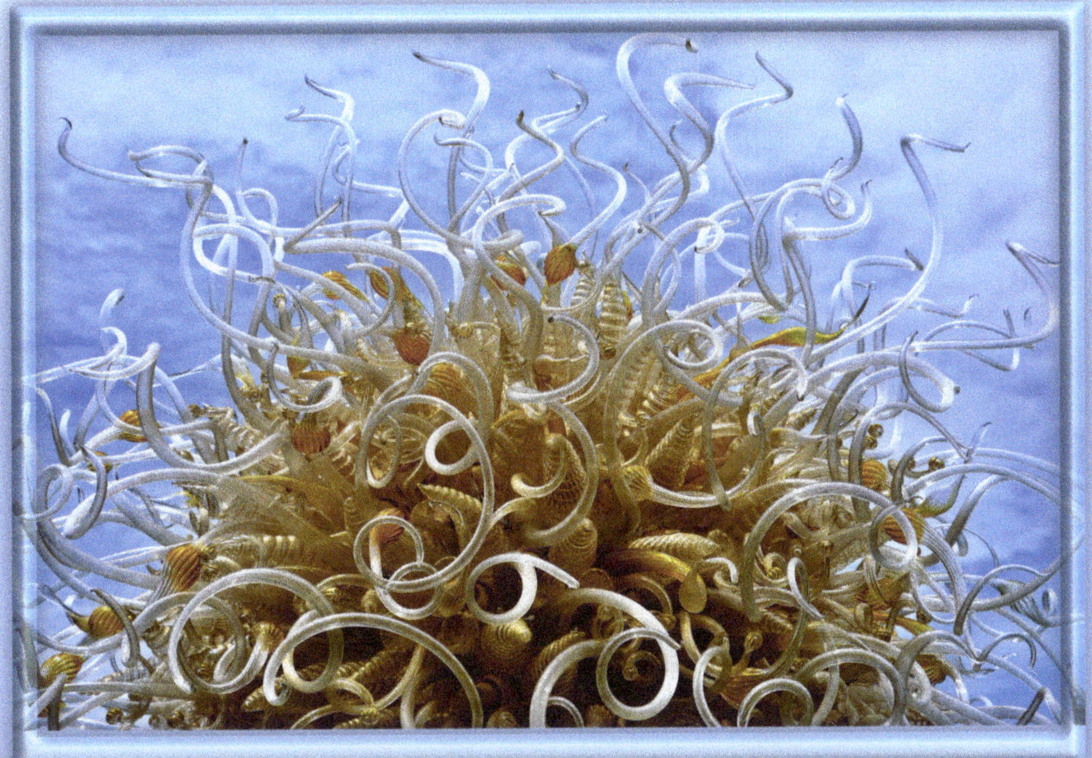

Certain Expectations

Things don't necessarily occur because we have expectations. Piaget noted that children have difficulty distinguishing between the objective and subjective in the world. Children sometimes believe their thoughts may directly make things happen - for instance, thinking harmful thoughts may cause your brother to trip on the steps and fall. Piaget coined this "magical thinking," and felt by age seven, children outgrew it. However, that is incorrect. Apparently, mainstream adults are continuing to engage in types of magical thinking. This is evidenced by the popular notion of The Law of Attraction, whose premise is that we attract events in our life with thoughts. For most, it can be difficult to imagine that anticipating an event will make it occur. The problem with certain expectations is that there needs to be a valid reason for the belief. If you believe that your expectations can bring you what you want without making any changes or effort toward it, you are using magical thinking and setting yourself up for some disappointment.[236]

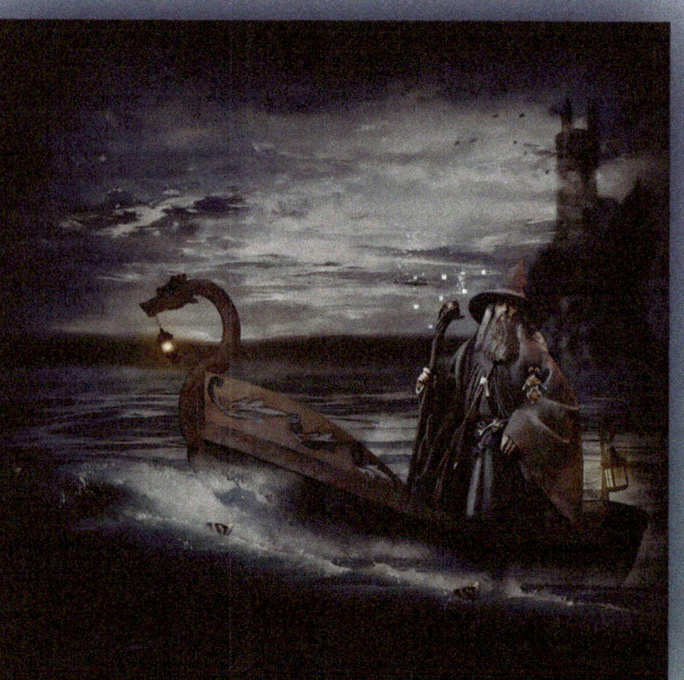

Courtesy of Marla Julien

Today I will evaluate whether I am a magical thinker. We have many reinforcements in our daily lives to support magical thinking. Journal about your expectations. What do you want to happen? Would you say your expectations are magical thinking, or are they realistic? Does magical thinking set you up for disappointment, or do you see it as a great coping mechanism? Is this an opportunity today to move into an adult thinking space? How do you feel about letting go of expectations? Sometimes in the workplace, certain expectations are required.

AUGUST 19

Day 231

Is Human Resources Your Friend?

The purpose of Human Resources (HR) is to protect companies from their employees, not to protect employees from companies. HR is supposed to preserve employee productivity by managing personnel problems. However, any protection employees receive is incidental because companies protect themselves through standard processes. Employees should not rely on the HR crew to protect them, defend them, or stick up for them unless aligning with the company's goal to protect itself from outside forces, including government regulations, public opinions, and the press.[244]

Today I will consider a time at work when I interacted with a Human Resources representative. Did it go as planned, or was the response opposite from what you expected? Journal about a time when you may not have received the support you needed. Or was there a time when you did receive the desired support from Human Resources?

Courtesy of Carrie Shank

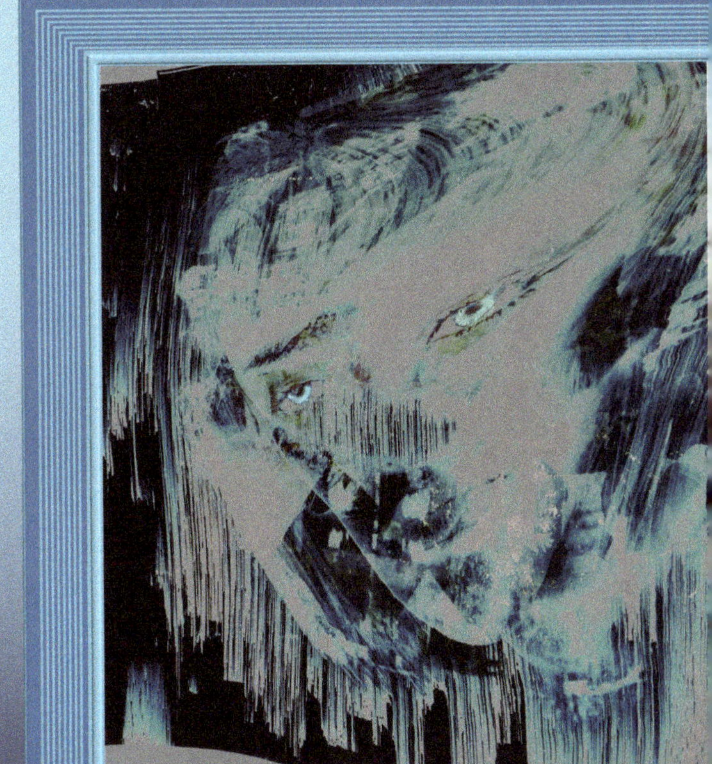

AUGUST 20

Day 232

Labeling People

Labeling people due to their behaviors and characteristics ends up hindering your curiosity about that person. Labeling may result in not exploring connections with people because you have certain ideas about them. Perhaps their beliefs are not in alignment with your own values. Imagine if others are labeling people constantly and do it to you. It would feel unfair, wouldn't it? We often do it to ourselves, unknowingly. There is a complex "hive of emotions," prior experiences, and a nuanced trail masked with every label. Labels result in conveying something complete, which is hard to veer from, once determined. "Why do this to yourself and prevent growth in other areas?"[245]

Courtesy of Nancy Nixon Ensign

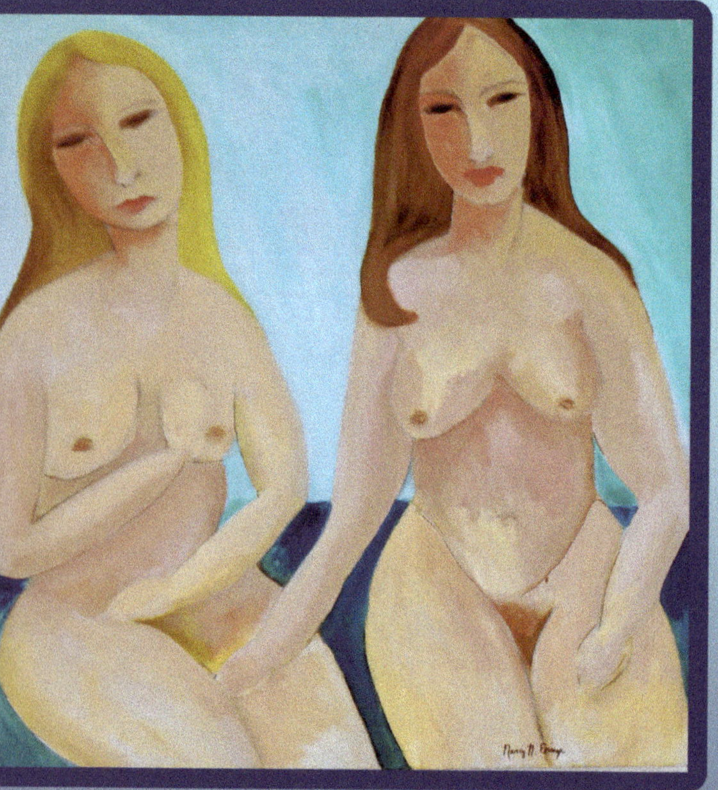

Today reflect on whether you have been labeled at home, in the community, or at work. Have you labeled others? Have you labeled yourself? Journal about the unfairness of having this done to you or others. Describe a time when labeling occurred. Think about some things you can do (and write a few down) to stop people from labeling each other and preventing growth.

AUGUST 21

Day 233

Think

"Be pleasant every morning until ten o' clock; the rest of the day will take care of itself."[246]

—W. Hunter & E. Hubbard

Today I will "think" about how setting the right tone for the day begins when I wake up and lasts until about 10 a.m. If you can remain pleasant until then, usually the rest of the day will continue in that direction. Think about a time when you woke up grouchy, and it ruined your whole day. Journal about the difference it makes when starting your day differently and what will typically follow after the morning hours set the tone. Think of a time when this made sense.

Courtesy of Umberto Kamperveen

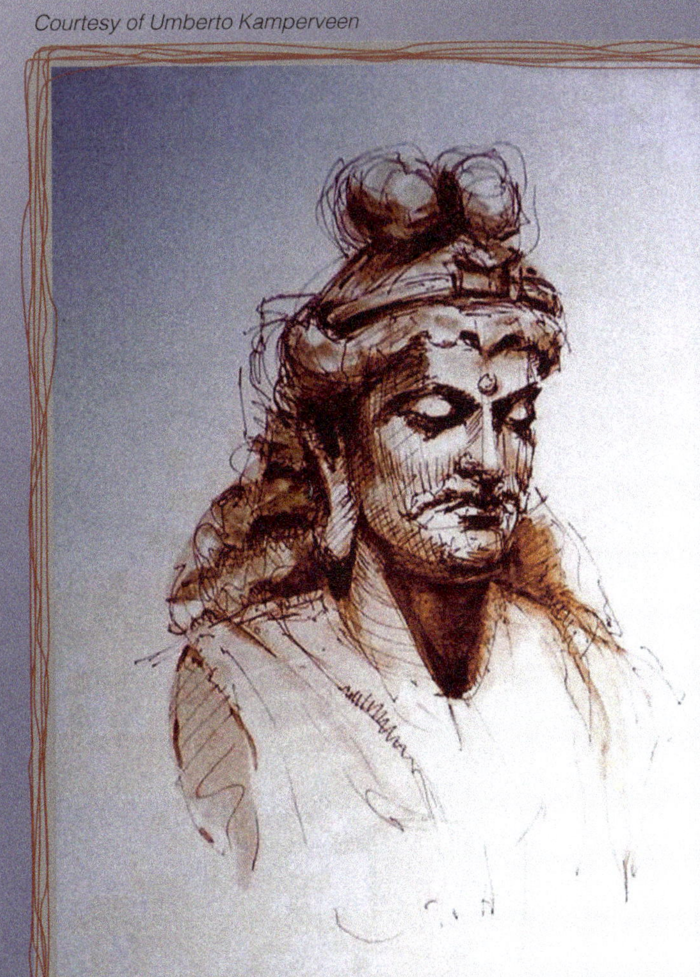

AUGUST 22

Day 234

Pandemic Traumatic Stress

Many people associate post-traumatic stress disorder (PTSD) with war. PTSD is a chronic disorder of the psyche that occurs with individuals having witnessed or experienced traumatic accidents, attacks, assaults, or other events. In 2003, healthcare workers and those who were quarantined had PTSD symptoms from the SARS outbreak. According to mental health experts, the Covid-19 pandemic may produce similar PTSD effects. Even without a diagnosis of PTSD, there may be strong, traumatic residual emotions that Covid-19 produces long after the pandemic.[247]

Today I will reflect on the time I spent social distancing and self-quarantining during the Covid-19 pandemic. Journal about how the pandemic personally affected you, the stress or PTSD that it caused, and how you chose to spend your time. Whether you are a hospital worker or any member of the community, have you been able to process everything and get support from any type of exposure or loss?

Courtesy of July Hodge

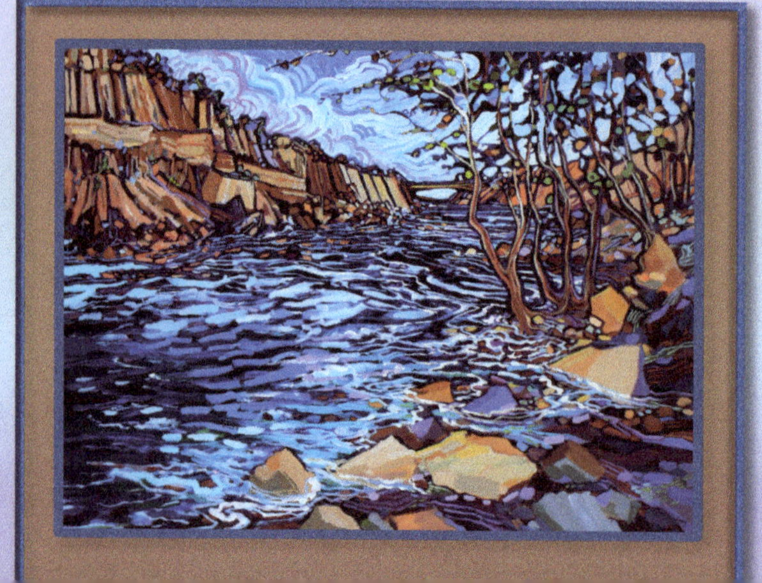

AUGUST 23

Day 235

Getting the Experience

Employers often state that there are plenty of educated applicants they can choose from, yet they are unable to find enough candidates who have on-the-job experience. Candidates report lengthy studying in addition to earning degrees, credentials, and certificates but are still unable to get jobs without actual work experience on their resume. Candidates also discuss how they worry that entry-level, service, hospitality, and retail jobs accessible to them may harm their chances of getting a position in their field, so they feel stuck.[248]

Today I will consider that finding a job, even though I have all the minimum qualifications listed in the employer's advertisement, is not as easy as I think. Maybe you have lots of experience but are looking to do a career transition. This can be even more difficult trying to break into something new without actual experience as a hiring requirement. Perhaps if organizations are having a difficult time finding someone with experience, they may be open to training, mentoring, or sponsoring a good candidate ready for advancement. Journal about a time when you applied for a job but didn't have the experience yet, and were offered the position. Think hard.

Courtesy of Rebecca Samler

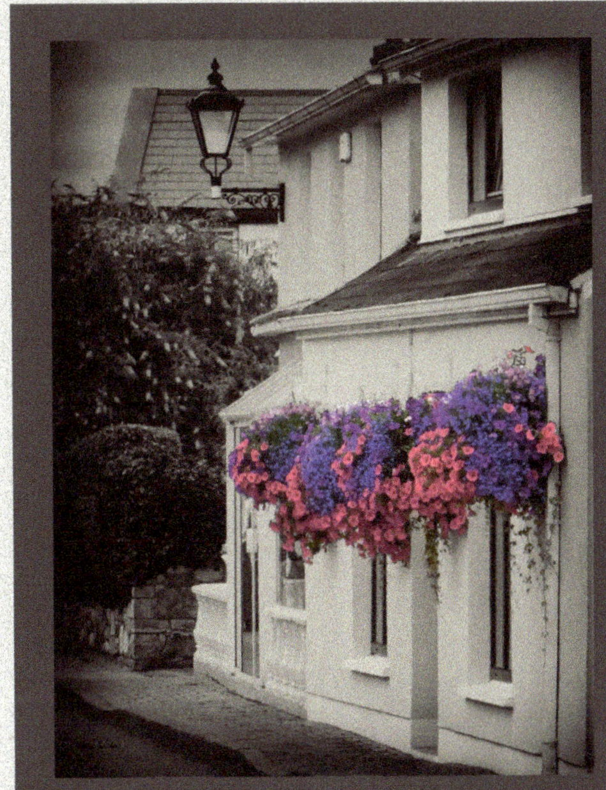

AUGUST 24

Day 236

Sound Judgment

We often think that our decisions are made with accurate facts. But everyone has unconscious biases affecting the choices they make. For instance, we may hire someone we are familiar with or who acts as we do. This keeps us away from unfamiliar territory or things we don't understand. Let's learn to arrive at sound judgments by filtering with wisdom and experience to reach thoughtful, smart decisions.[249]

Today I will consider if my judgment is sound. Whether you are in a management or staff position, journal about your experience with making decisions. Making important decisions can be stressful. Are your decisions free of explicit and implicit biases? Describe a recent decision that you needed to make and how you went about it. Did you base that decision on being objective or subjective?

Courtesy of Susan Gutierrez

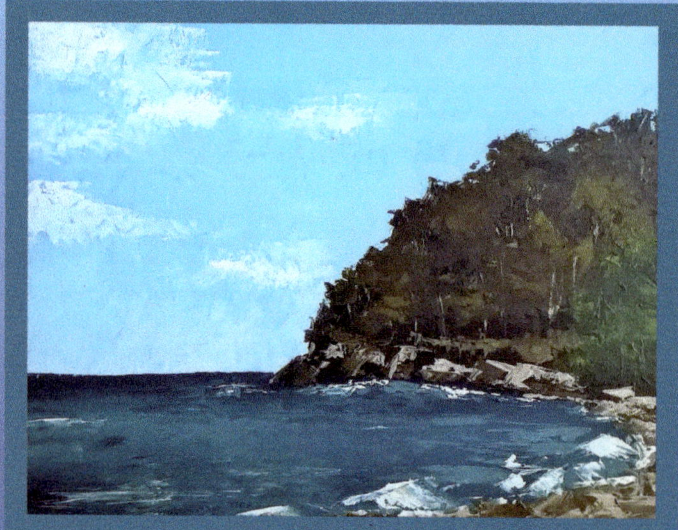

Quitting

AUGUST

25

Day 237

Having a shortage of PPE nationwide, and being required to reuse the same mask and gown the whole shift, has been unfortunate. Most can agree we do not think it is safe. Before the pandemic, we did not reuse. If we entered a room, left, and had to return, we used a new gown and mask before going back in. "I reacted out of stress and fear because of not having the protective gear." Quitting was necessary because "I have no one else to care for my children if something happens to me."[250]

Today I will reflect on whether I have ever quit a job. Journal about this experience. How did you go about doing it? Did you give proper notice? Was your decision based on "flight or fight," excessive stress, workload, fatigue, personal safety, cynicism, or perhaps depersonalization? When a job puts your life at risk due to failures from above, is quitting legitimate?

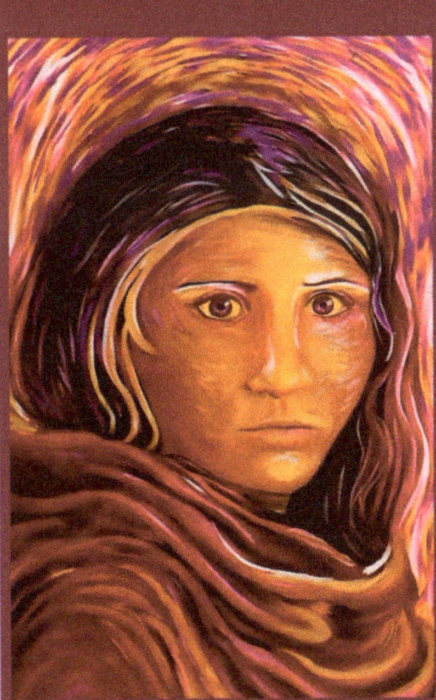

Courtesy of Jill Mattson

AUGUST 26

Day 238

Progress and AI

Machine algorithms that learn are beginning to overtake human performance with many specific and some narrow sectors that involve medical diagnoses and image recognition. They are also swiftly progressing in more intricate domains, such as creating eerie texts mimicking human communication (chatbots). We are progressively relying on machine algorithms for making decisions with broad topics. The topics range from tracking what people spend time observing to who will get certain jobs. But we are unable to explain how the machine algorithms arrive at the choices they make. How can we legitimize placing responsibility on these computer systems? Should machine learning algorithms make decisions affecting peoples' lives if we can't comprehend how those decisions were made?[251]

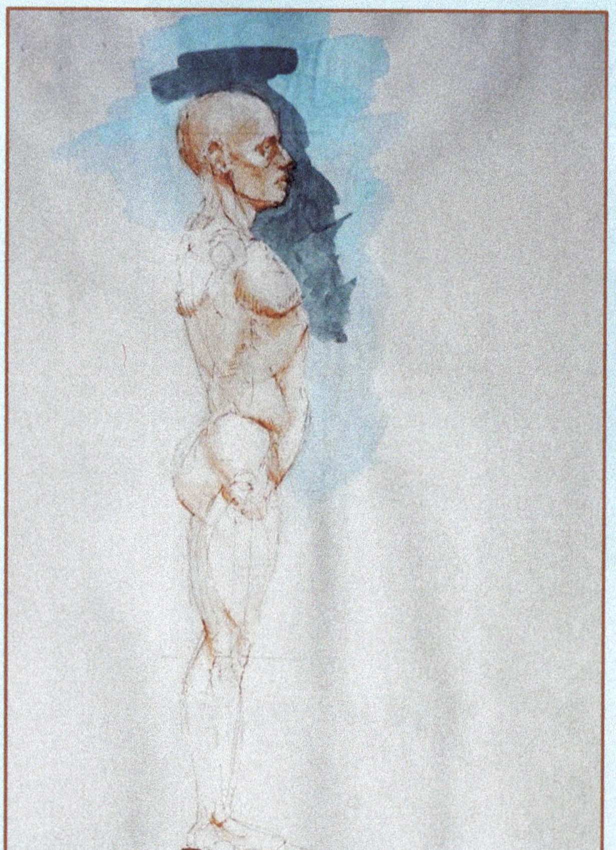

Courtesy of Umberto Kamperveen

Today I will consider artificial intelligence and the impact it has on our daily lives. Can you journal about how progress and artificial intelligence has either improved or decreased satisfaction at work or your home life? When AI isn't performing what is intended, this can create stress for all parties.

AUGUST 27

Day 239

Relaxing your Mind

There are many ways for you to relax. Some methods are designed for calming your mind, while some are for relaxing your body. However, since the body and mind are connected, many methods of relaxation are designed for both.[252]

Today is another opportunity to remind myself to practice self-care. You may be dieting, exercising, and taking good care of your body now. However, taking care of your mind and experiencing deep relaxation is essential for having harmony in your life. Journal about your self-care activities (besides journaling) and the mind/body relaxation methods you are using daily.

Courtesy of Ann Parker

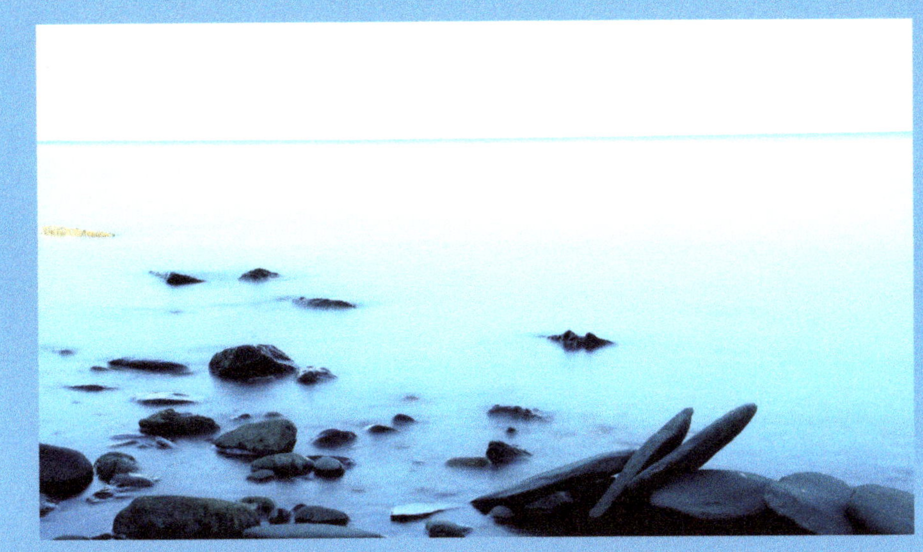

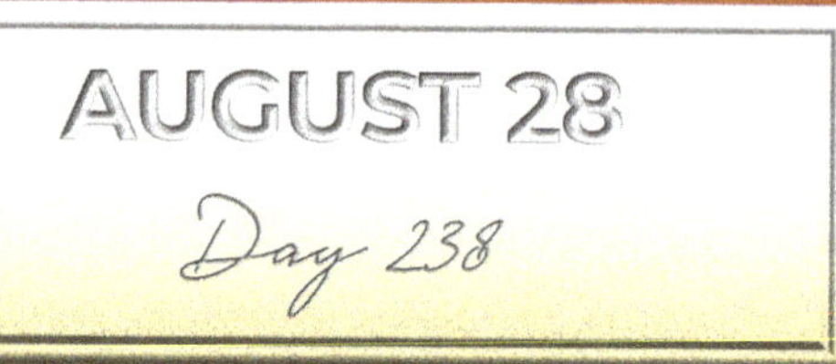

Your Critical Inner Voice

Your critical inner voice acts as an enemy, which can affect all aspects of your life. This includes your confidence and self-esteem, intimate and personal relationships, and accomplishments and performances at work, school, and home. These pessimistic thoughts can affect you by undermining positive thoughts about yourself and others. These feelings also foster self-criticism, distrust, inwardness, addictions, self-denial, and withdrawal from goal-oriented activities.[253]

Courtesy of Kevin Dunne

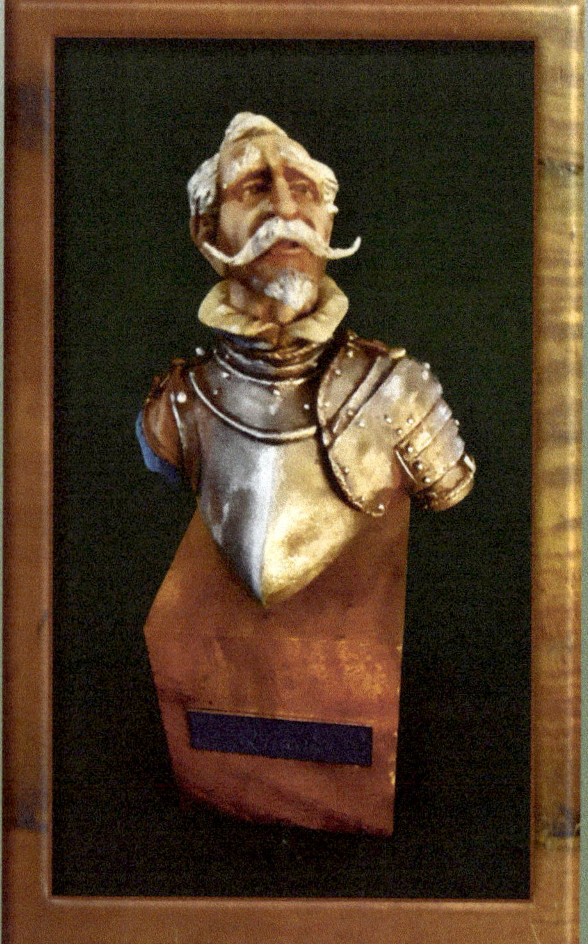

Today I will consider my critical inner voice that can affect so many aspects of my life. Journal about your critical inner voice. Describe how it behaves and the things it tells you. Are these things true, or are they negative? Do they inhibit you from achieving whatever goals you may set for yourself? Can you learn how to stop these thoughts and cognitively restructure your critical inner voice? It takes practice and conscientiousness. Does your critical inner voice create stress for you?

AUGUST 29

Day 241

Nurturing Your Spirit

We are in an era of accessible information filled with opportunities that absorb our energy and time. Now and then, we may feel that anguish in our souls to seek higher meaning and listen to our inner voice, saying to us, "be still." Acquiring the spirituality for exploring, getting adequate rest, using meditation, mindfulness, and deep breathing can be vital. Also, having gratitude, choosing to forgive, maintaining positive relationships, or going on a nature walk can all be good ways of nurturing your spirit.[254]

Today I will journal about how I nurture my spirit. Reflect on what things you have done this week that are listed above. If you haven't done anything from the list, what things can you plan to do? Since starting the journal, you have kept up with your self-care. By doing so, you can "be still" and nurture your spirit.

Courtesy of Judy Hodge

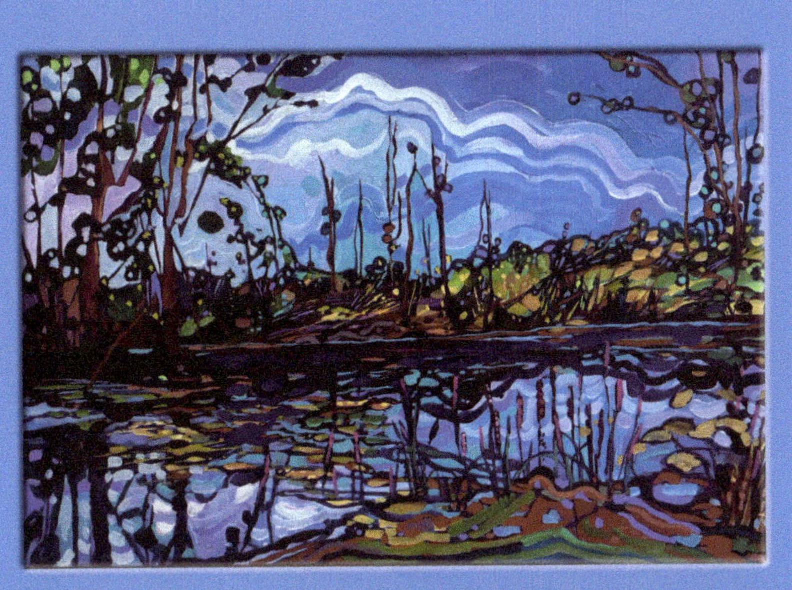

AUGUST 30

Day 242

Getting Enough Sleep

Think you are getting enough sleep? Those that are experiencing burnout may have trouble falling asleep since they are ruminating about work. Even when you do drift asleep, it's typical for your rest to be undermined and broken. Are you often waking up in the morning still exhausted?[255]

Today I will evaluate my sleep pattern. In your journal, describe the past month and how you have slept. Can you rate your sleep pattern on a scale of 1-10, with 10 being the best and 1 being the worst? How would you rate the quality of your sleep? What other symptoms do you experience if you have sleeplessness? Do you sleep too much or not enough? What do you believe is affecting your sleep pattern? Sleepfoundation.org has sleep hygiene tips online. Which ones can you commit to?

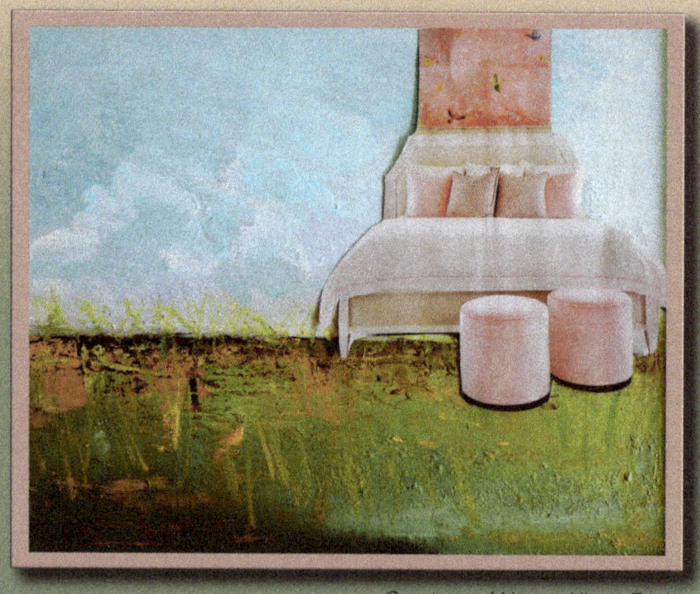

Courtesy of Nancy Nixon Ensign

AUGUST 31 Day 243

Chore Wars

Are chore wars over housework trivial? Once you start tracking how much time you are spending doing housework, you might be shocked at the actual amount of hours. Sometimes women may have extra household responsibilities. Sometimes men use their free time recharging while advancing their careers. Sometimes women may lose track of their priorities, not moving ahead with things of importance to them. Have men figured it out? Many men aren't exactly raising hands, volunteering to do more housework. American men do more household chores than prior decades but are they doing as many household chores as women?[256]

Today I will reflect on the chores at home and the stress and exhaustion they create. Journal about your chores and how they may be inhibiting you from advancing your other goals. Make a list of all the chores that you perform in the household. Then, make a list of the chores that your significant other performs. Is it balanced? If not, what is your plan to eliminate your stress and exhaustion for potentially overcompensating? Is there a certain stereotype in your household regarding roles and chores?

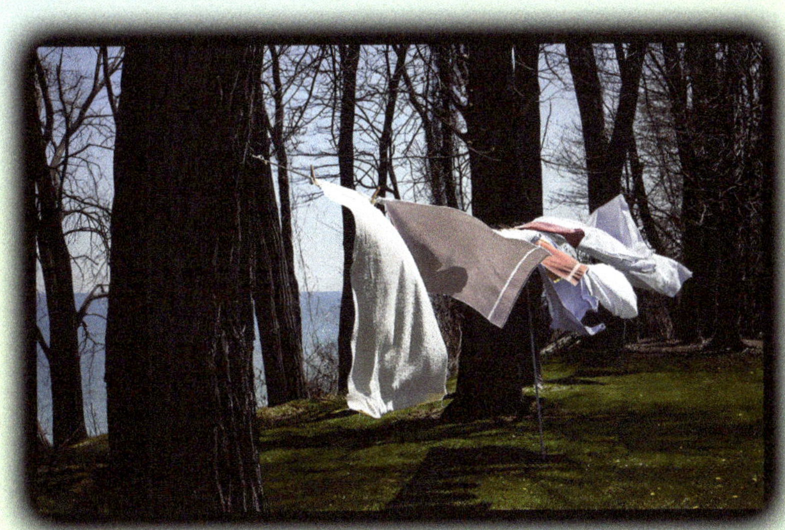

Courtesy of Rebecca Samler

SEPTEMBER 1

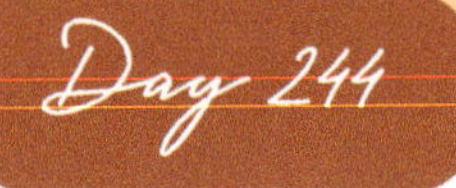

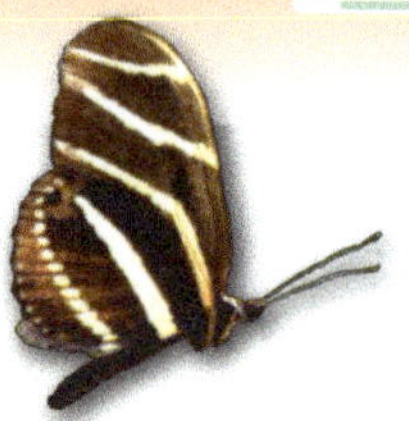

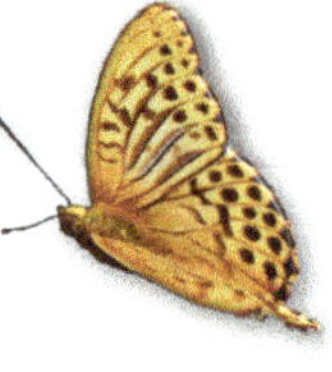

Achieving

When achieving your most aspirational goals and then sitting back, propping up your feet, and no longer pushing yourself, you may become directionless and lost.[257]

Today I will think about everything I have achieved and things that I still want to accomplish. Journal about three major things you have achieved in the past five years and three things you would like to achieve in the upcoming five years. If you haven't set any goals for your future, start today. Use the creative side of your brain and imagine yourself already finishing those goals. What does the end result look like?

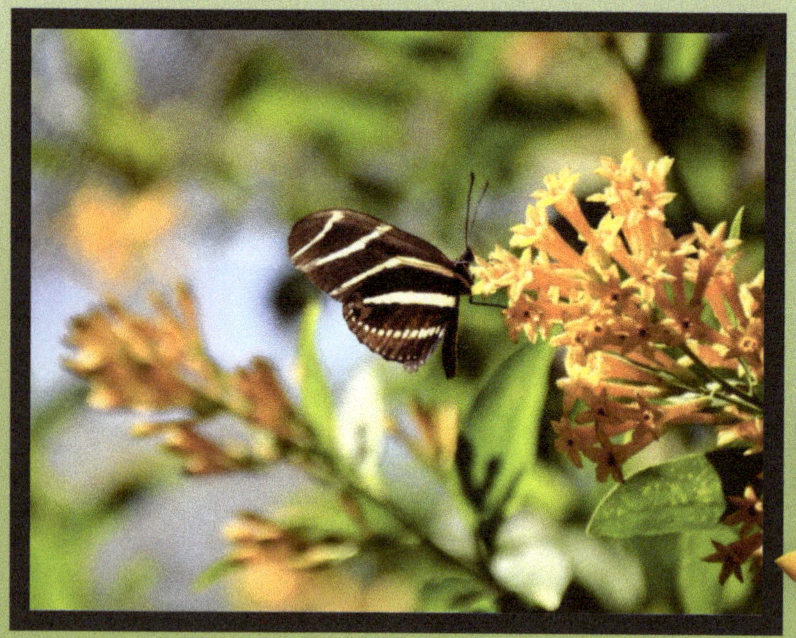

Courtesy of Linda Probst

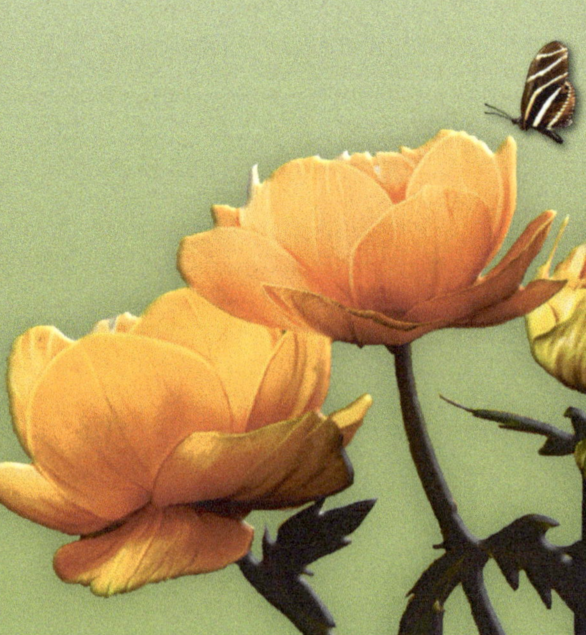

SEPTEMBER 2

Day 245

Misinformation

There is an endless plethora of political misinformation, many with bold lies that are inescapable online. We are living in a world with truth challenges.[258]

Today I will consider how misinformation and disinformation impact my daily life via the media and social media. Has your interpretation of reality caused strife between family, friends, or coworkers because of the information you choose to believe? Journal about how you go about seeking trustworthy resources for the consumption of the news you follow.

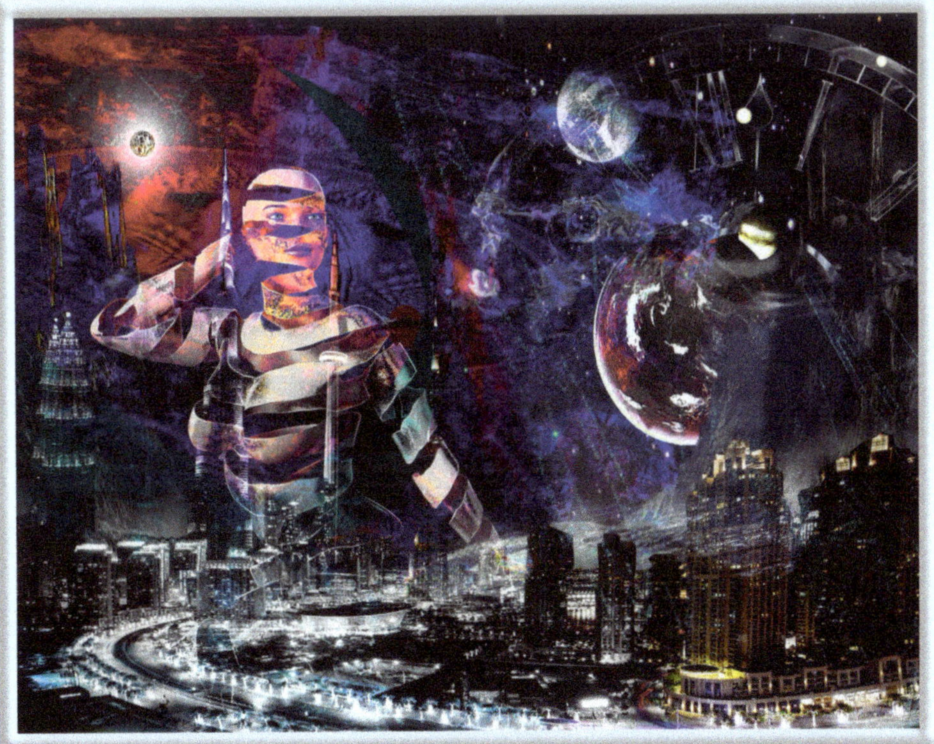

Courtesy of Carrie Shank

SEPTEMBER 3

Day 246

Leveraging

When having the "upper hand," a person is using what is known as leverage. Experience and knowledge may help you achieve a certain position. Exclusivity in specific markets, reducing product pricing, improving service options, and delivering value in your personal relationships (emphasize "personal") is how you leverage.[259]

Today I will consider the influence I have, even though I may not be in a leadership role. Journal about how you can use your informal power to leverage things you want both at home and in the workplace for your client or yourself. It is not wrong to leverage and know your value. Describe the ways you engage in personal relationships that make the ability to leverage possible. Leveraging can be altruistic and not necessarily self-serving.

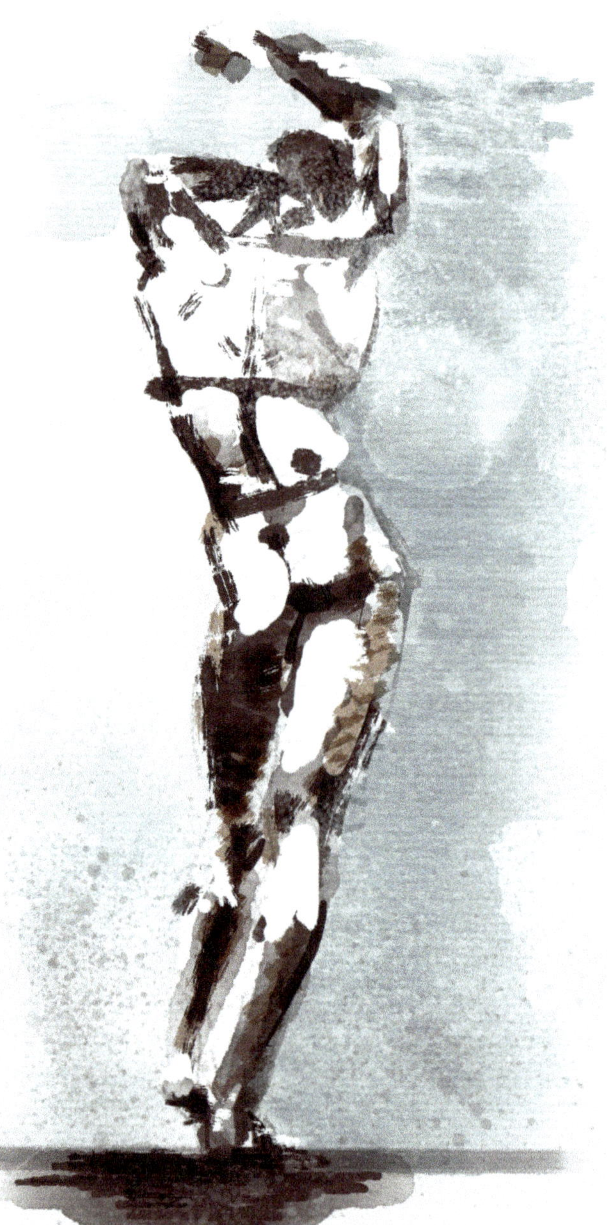

Courtesy of Umberto Kamperveen

SEPTEMBER 4

Day 247

The Neighborhood

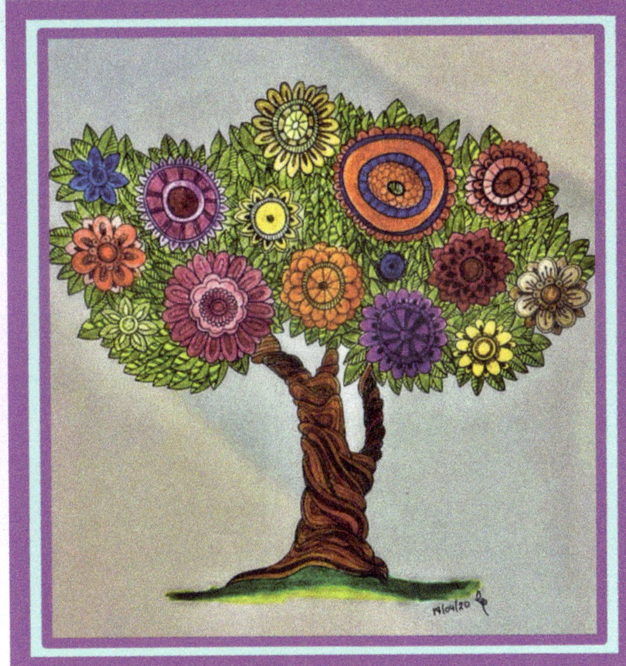
Courtesy of Eduardo Andres

Neighborhood context can affect psychological wellbeing. Living in an adverse neighborhood may create a greater stress load, increase reactivity to life events, and harm the quality of social relationships. Personality traits allow one to adjust and moderate the impact neighborhoods have on psychological wellbeing. Some people who have particularly strong personalities can cope effectively with neighborhood stressors, while others end up significantly mentally harmed.[260]

Today I will consider the neighborhood I live and work in. Journal about each neighborhood you've lived in and the impact it had on your wellbeing. Describe your neighborhoods by making two lists with five adjectives each. Examine the words in your list for each column. What does each column of adjectives present? Describe your impressions from the exercise.

SEPTEMBER 5

Day 248

Being Reasonable

When making a mistake, prepare to own accountability. Many parents know the dilemma of an irksome unaccountable offspring. The glass cookie jar suddenly shatters in your kitchen. You rush in to find your kid, standing alone, telling you, "I didn't do it!" Really? Being reasonable, we realize that owning up to a mistake will solve the problem most of the time. When you don't, it sparks and ignites the problem, which may be uncontainable later. Don't make excuses when realizing it's your team that has dropped the ball.[261]

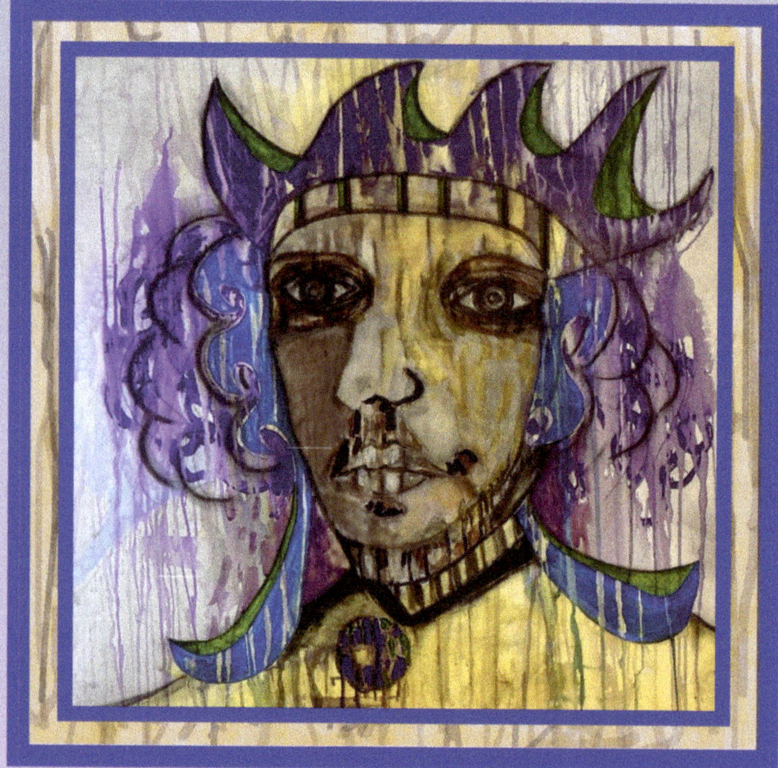

Courtesy of Edward Berkise

Today I will consider whether I find myself being reasonable. There is no perfect human being. Journal about a time you took accountability when you realized you dropped the ball. What was the last cookie jar that you shattered? How was your apology received? What did you learn from your humility? Standing all alone to assume responsibility might be irksome, but if addressed quickly, it may fix or contain a very large problem.

SEPTEMBER 6

Day 249

Reflecting

Reflection is a method of examining and exploring ourselves, our attributes, perspectives, actions, interactions, and experiences. Reflecting helps us gain insight and see how we can move forward. Its power is in developing our understanding of the ways we learn, the topics we study, and defining our long-term goals. Reflecting can help promote problem-solving skills and critical thinking.[262]

Today I will reflect on a recent stressful interaction with a coworker, boss, spouse, friend, or child. Journal about the insight you reached from reflecting about the way you behaved. What was your reaction? Was the reaction you had ideal? When you reflect, write about alternative reactions to perfect for the next time.

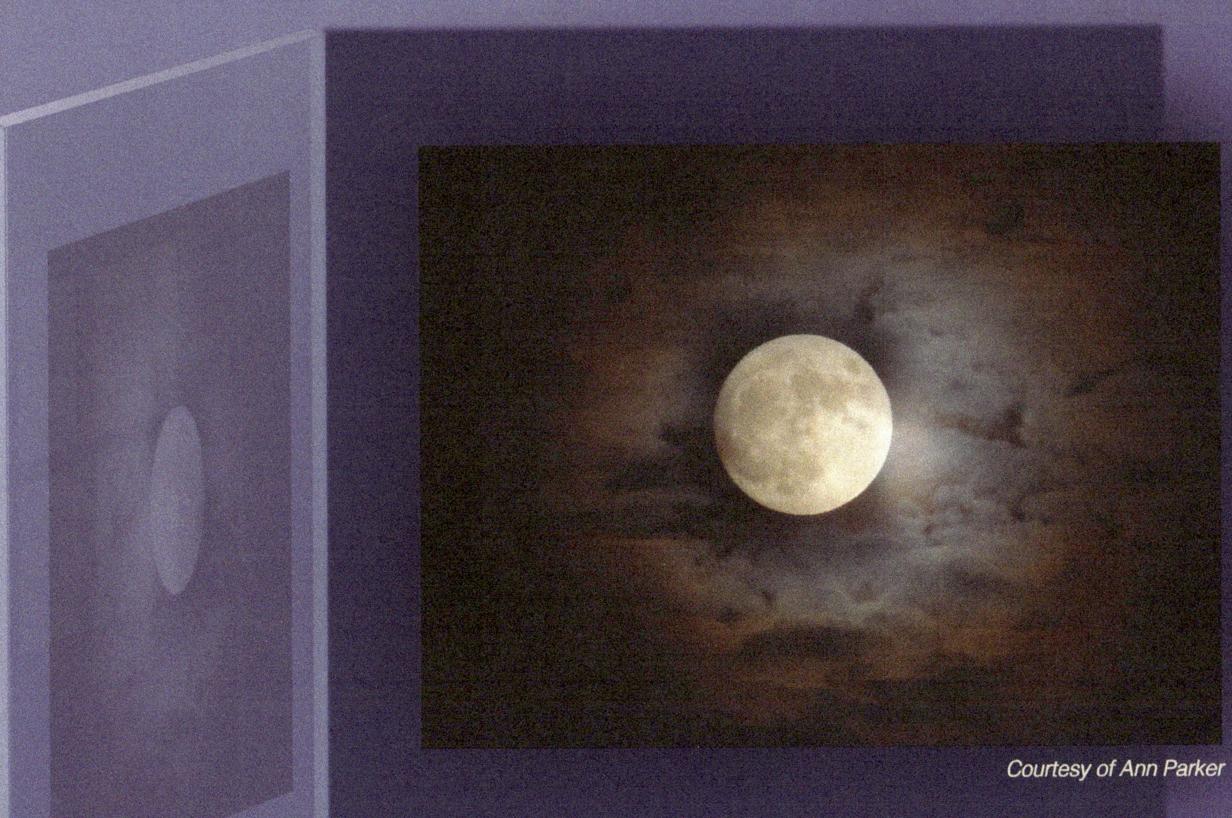

Courtesy of Ann Parker

SEPTEMBER 7 *Day 250*

Less is More

In a 19th century poem by Robert Browning, printed in Andrea del Sarto, the phrase "less is more" was first found in print. It reads:

> "Who strive - you don't know how the others strive
> To paint a little thing like that you smeared
> Carelessly passing with your robes afloat -
> Yet do much less, so much less, Someone says,
> (I know his name, no matter) - so much less!
> Well, less is more, Lucrezia."[263]

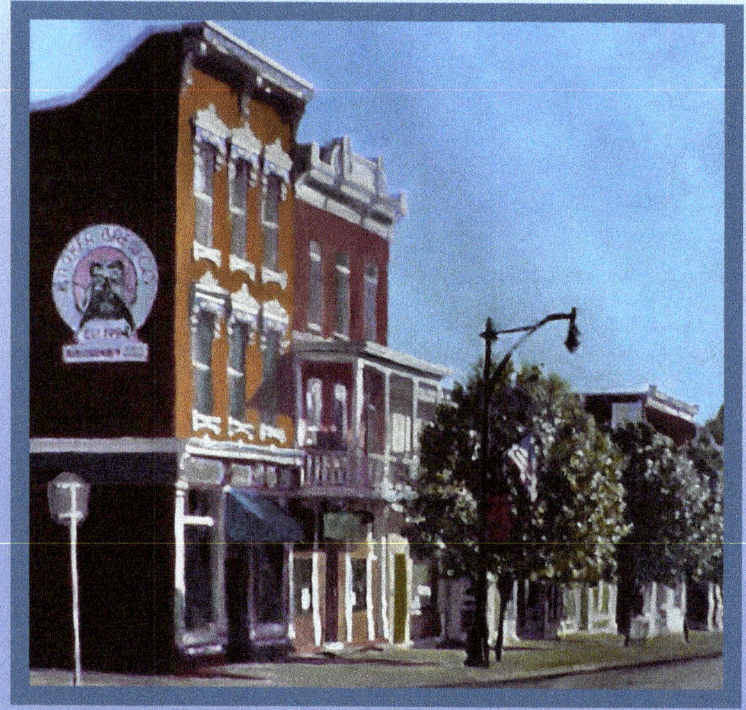

Courtesy of Susan MacKay

Today I will consider how often excessiveness can bring about stress. Learning to keep things simple and minimal can be beneficial in creating less confusion. Journal about a time you simplified a process. How did you benefit from simplifying? Write about an instance where less was more. Reflect.

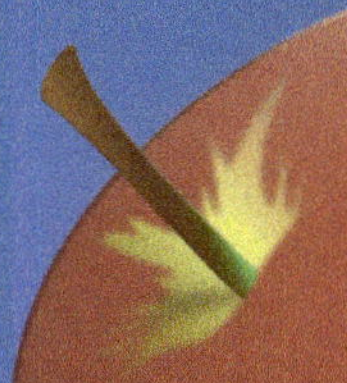

SEPTEMBER 8

Day 251

Banding Together

Generations to come must be able to rely on the future of agricultural sustainability without compromise. It is important to have equal consideration of short and long-term stewardship that promotes natural, human, and economic prosperity. To be a good steward, the health and safety of consumers, laborers, and those working and living in rural communities, now and in the future, must be considered. Stewardship includes maintaining the quality of the land and our natural resources in a way that regenerates them in the future. Animal welfare is also a great concern, particularly the care of livestock and farming enterprises. Over the past 40 years, many questions about high costs have initiated growing movements for emerging innovations. Increasing support and movements for acceptance of sustainable agriculture is necessary for protecting and conserving safe food production. Environmental health, social equity, and economic profitability are three objectives for sustainable agriculture.[264]

Today I will consider how banding together for healthcare, economic stability, agricultural and environmental purity, and social justice can make policy change. Journal about one of these stress-inducing issues mentioned where you banded with others to create influence for an issue important to you. How did this benefit you and the group? Banding together can be exhausting (for introverts), but when there is a common purpose, it can be quite effective for reaching goals.

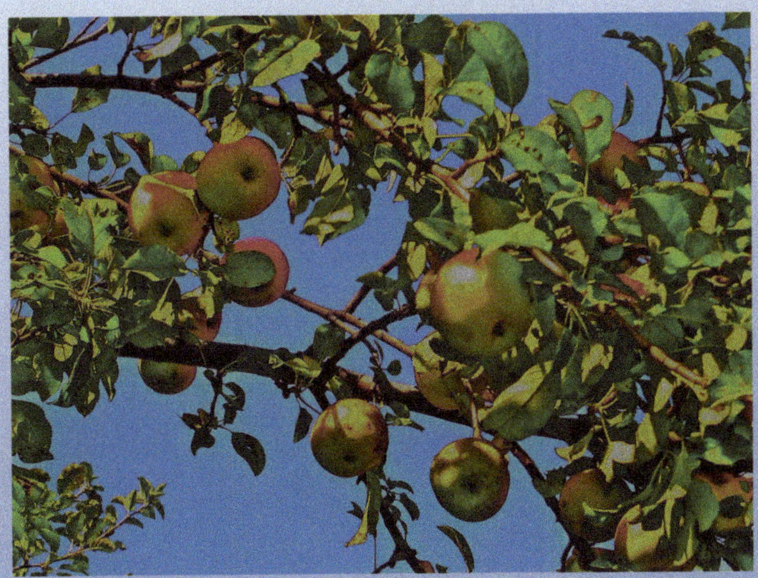

Courtesy of Robert John Holland

SEPTEMBER 9

Day 252

Cliques at Work

Excessive togetherness, aka "cliques," can be harmful to companies since those who are left out become dissatisfied and distracted within their work environments. Employees may exhaust more energy attempting to find coping mechanisms to counter the cliques rather than put forth effort into their jobs. Cliques cause staff to focus on fitting into certain groups rather than actual work and the company. This impacts an organization's bottom line. It can also cause good workers to leave the company once enough is enough.[265]

Today I will evaluate the cliques within my workplace. Are you part of a clique or on the outside? Journal about what you have witnessed regarding cliques at work and whether you contribute to or act against cliques in the workplace. Cliques are not inclusive and perpetuate homogeneity or uniformity. When teammates are not included, this is stressful, disrespectful, and can lead to burnout.

Courtesy of Rebecca Samler

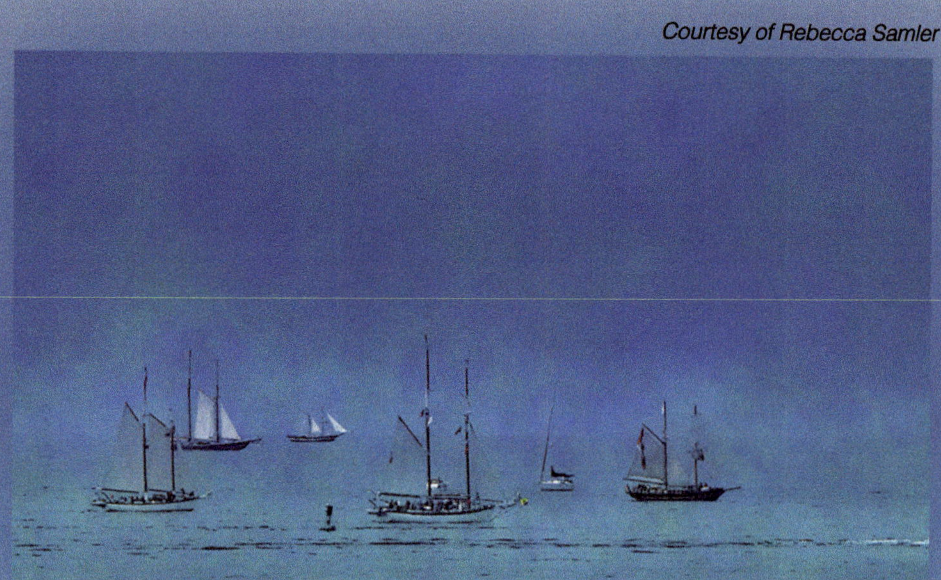

Faster, Hurry

People with a forceful "hurry-up" drive tend to be perfectionists who prefer being in control. These people have been raised to believe in a clear right or wrong way of handling situations. They feel that other solutions are flawed or of lesser value. These personalities often hate to stray from their routine behaviors, whether traveling, cooking, or working. They rarely use other methods to achieve what they want to accomplish. They have been taught to finish everything quickly and that asking for help or admitting to being overworked or overloaded indicates weakness. Their only solution is always to hurry. When we constantly operate at a maximum rate, we signal a physiological communication causing adrenaline to rush and cortisol to surge. This causes anxiousness, impatience, irritability, or nausea. We are more likely to forget and overlook things when we operate too quickly and don't take sufficient time, which is how mistakes happen.[266]

Today I will think about whether I am the type of person to hurry and rush through my projects. Journal about the pace at which you normally operate. Rate your speed when performing tasks. If you perform things quickly, rate yourself as a 1, and rate yourself a 10 if you operate thoroughly and methodically at a reasonable pace. How does your pace contribute to stress, work overload, cynicism, fatigue, moral distress, and ultimately burnout?

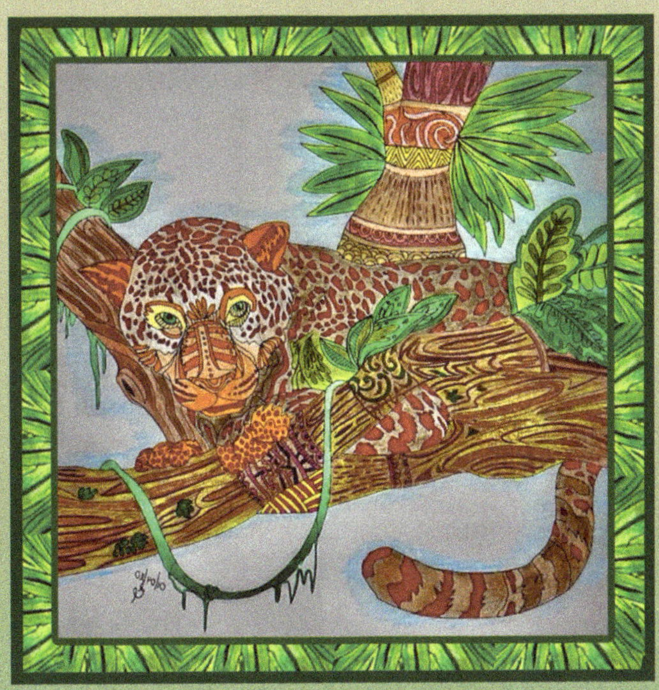

Courtesy of Eduardo Andres

SEPTEMBER 11

Day 254

Remembrance

Here we are, many years have passed, and newer generations that weren't born or were too young are unable to remember the unthinkable terrorist attacks on The World Trade Center. They learn secondhand how horrifying September 11, 2001, was for so many. Remembering the 9/11 events doesn't become easier.[267]

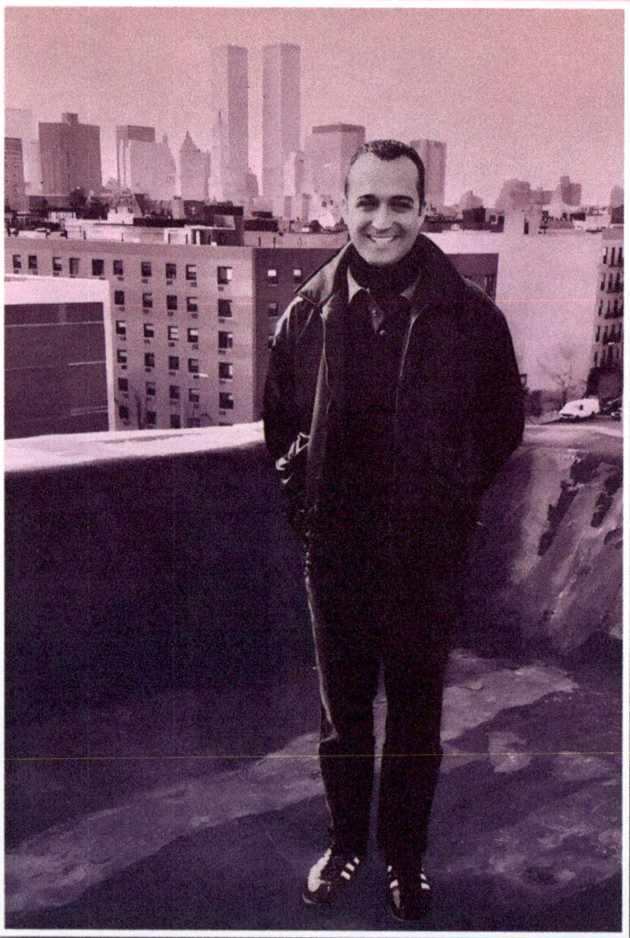

Courtesy of Umberto Kamperveen

Today I will begin with a moment of remembrance for the victims of 9/11, their families, and loved ones. Journal about where you were on 9/11 if you were even born. An entire generation has passed. It is an important event to remember so that similar events can be prevented, if possible. In your journal, describe your flashback when you first learned of the 9/11 attacks. The stress and trauma the entire nation and world felt will never be forgotten.

My Home Environment

There are proactive steps to avoid injury and disease. Maintaining a healthy environment at home is crucial as preventive medicine for you and your family. A healthy emotional environment is needed for a sound, healthy home. Family members that communicate effectively are willing to settle and resolve conflicts. Doing so fosters wellbeing.[268]

Today I will consider my home environment. Journal about what it is like living in your house. Discuss how your home environment impacts your performance at work. What three things do you enjoy the most about your home environment, and what three things would you like to change the most about it? If wanting changes at home, what new outcomes would you like to see?

Courtesy of Nancy Nixon Ensign

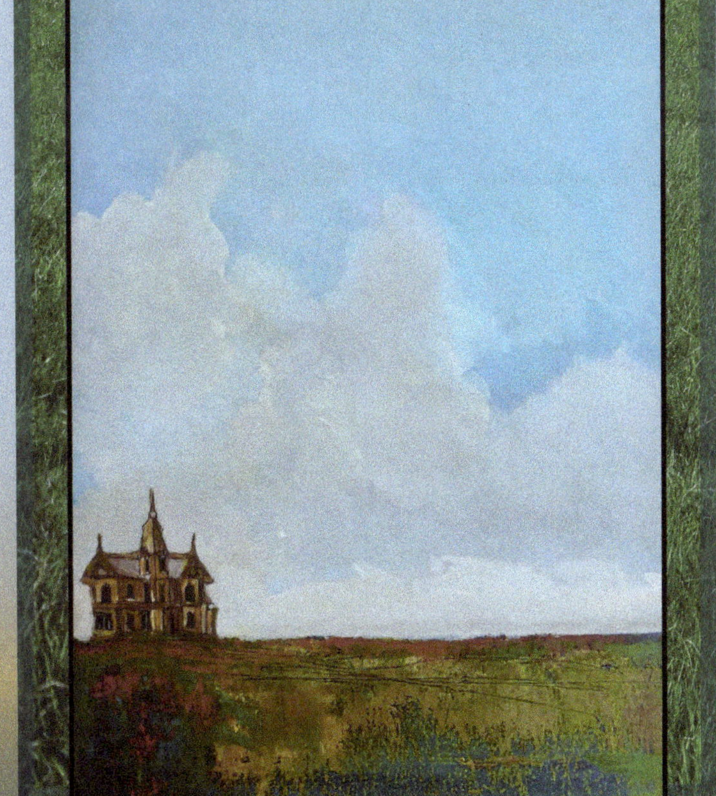

SEPTEMBER 13

Day 256

Abundance of Caution

An "abundance of caution" is a phrase most of us have heard. There are different subtleties, but the gist is to be extra careful. What situations are applicable? It is mostly when there is a remote possibility of a disaster when risks and benefits are not measured correctly. Caution is not a proper remedy for not knowing the facts.[269] As effortlessly as "abundance of caution" rolls off our tongue, it acts as a kind of doublespeak. In the case of the pandemic, the phrase may stimulate tranquility, assuming hunkering down may be a pleasure that can be enjoyed by all. However, many people are unable to afford activities for the sake of caution. Some Americans are emptying the shelves at the grocery store, while others are enduring restrictions placed on food stamp assistance.[270]

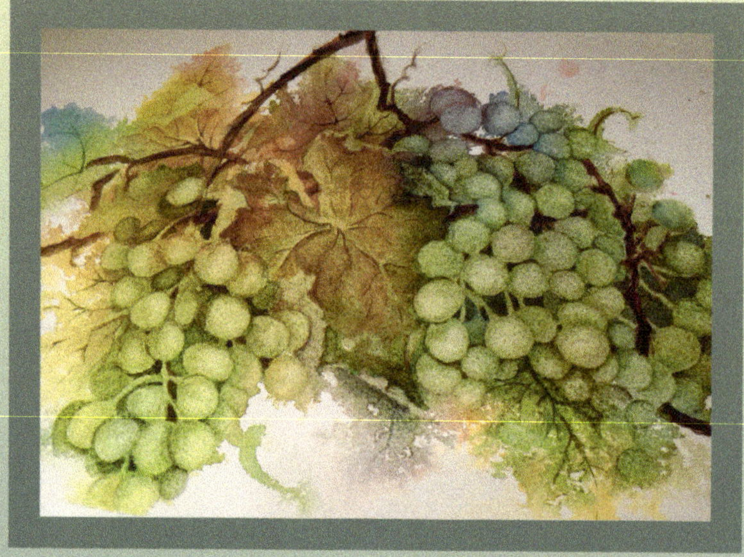

Courtesy of Ronnie Lafferty

Today I will consider abundance - mine and others. When there is a lack of abundance, how does that impact stress levels? Journal about whether abundance is evident at home, or the contrary. Describe a time when you used an abundance of caution at work or home to measure the risk versus benefit of something important. Notice the difference in abundance and having caution.

SEPTEMBER 14

Day 257

Social Media and Burnout

When you take a vacation from using social media, it doesn't mean that you no longer care. It simply means that you understand your limits and need time to replenish. When you don't make mental wellbeing your top priority, it makes other situations in life difficult. Be sure to question whether your social media posts are making a positive impact. Does your social media make you a change agent? Is it healthy to vent online, or does it generate arguments with others that seem unending? If you discover social media is draining your energy, it may be a good time to take a break and assess the role it holds in your daily life and the way you choose to handle it.[271]

Today I will consider my use of social media. Journal about your social media habits. Have you had any Facebook or Instagram fights recently? Has someone blocked you, or you blocked them because the communication was ineffective and oppositional? Ask yourself if social media is entirely healthy or causing stress, unnecessary anxiety, anger, or frustration. What other things could you be doing besides social media? What things could you be developing?

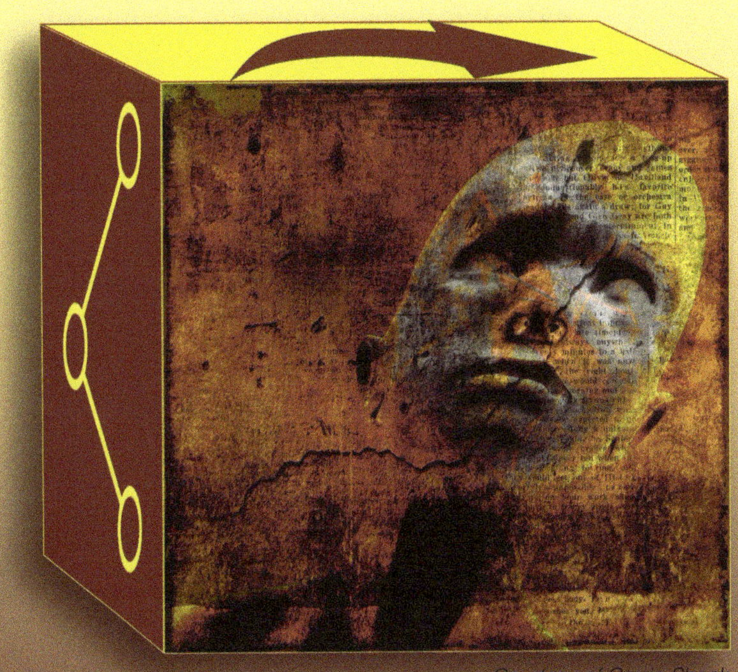

Courtesy of Carrie Shank

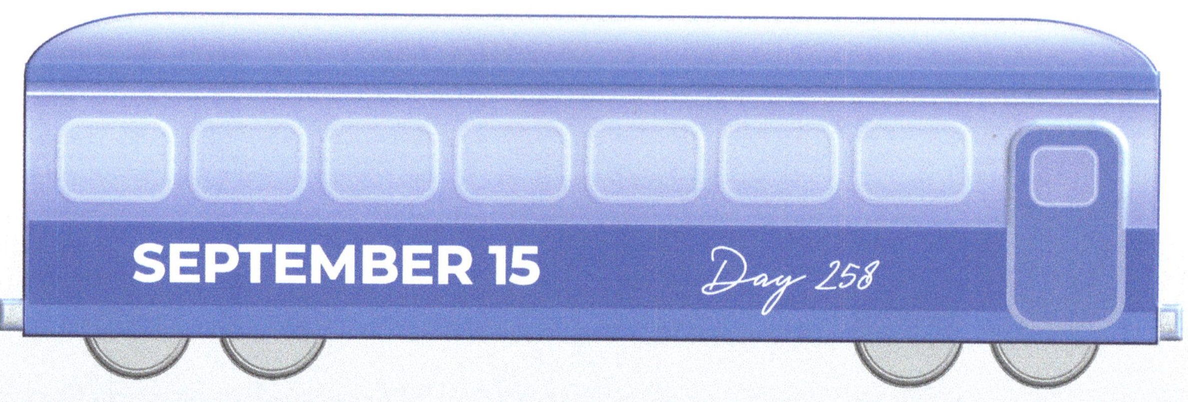

Derailment

To stave off derailment, a word of advice would be to enhance your sense of self-awareness. Knowing your strengths and your weaknesses helps leaders understand themselves - as well as how others view them. Often, derailed leaders do not understand until it is too late that they did not fit in well, their leadership style was not working with the job demands, and the direction they were going in was not aligned with the organization's path. Certain situations trigger derailment that managers should be alert to, such as boredom, careers in transition, and work overload.[272]

Today I will think about a time when I may have been derailed. Certain leadership styles may not work. For those that are not aware of how others perceive them, derailment may be imminent. Journal about a time where work overload, career transitions, or boredom were at stake. What happened? What role did you play in the derailment? If you were derailed, how did you overcome the occurrence? Write down your advice for others about derailment.

Courtesy of Lisa Schultz

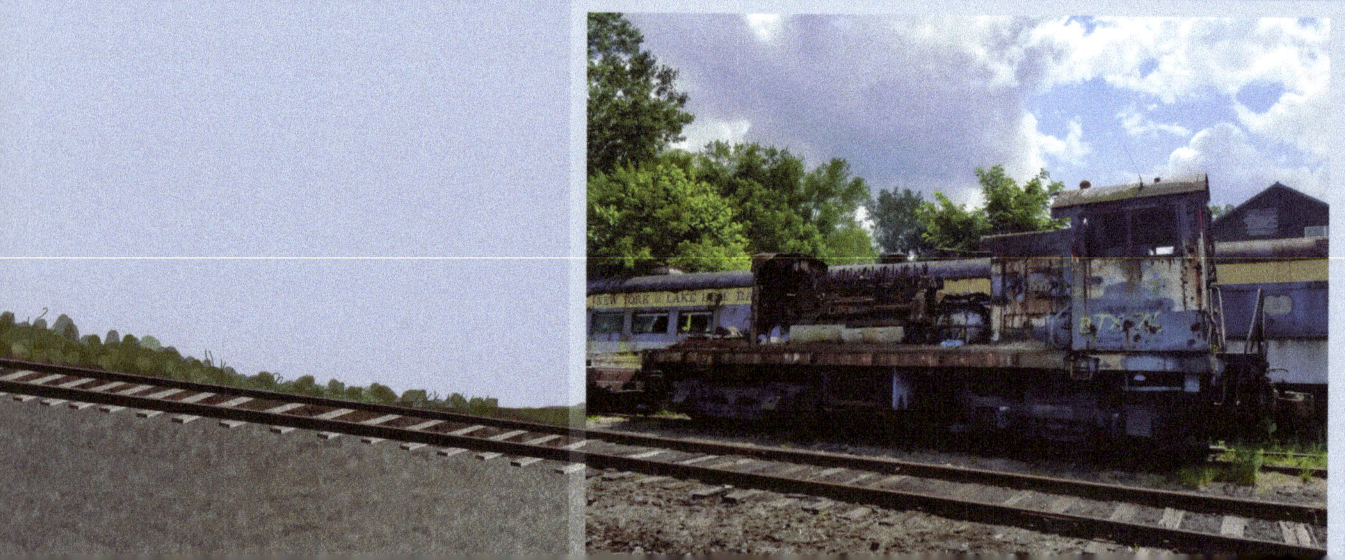

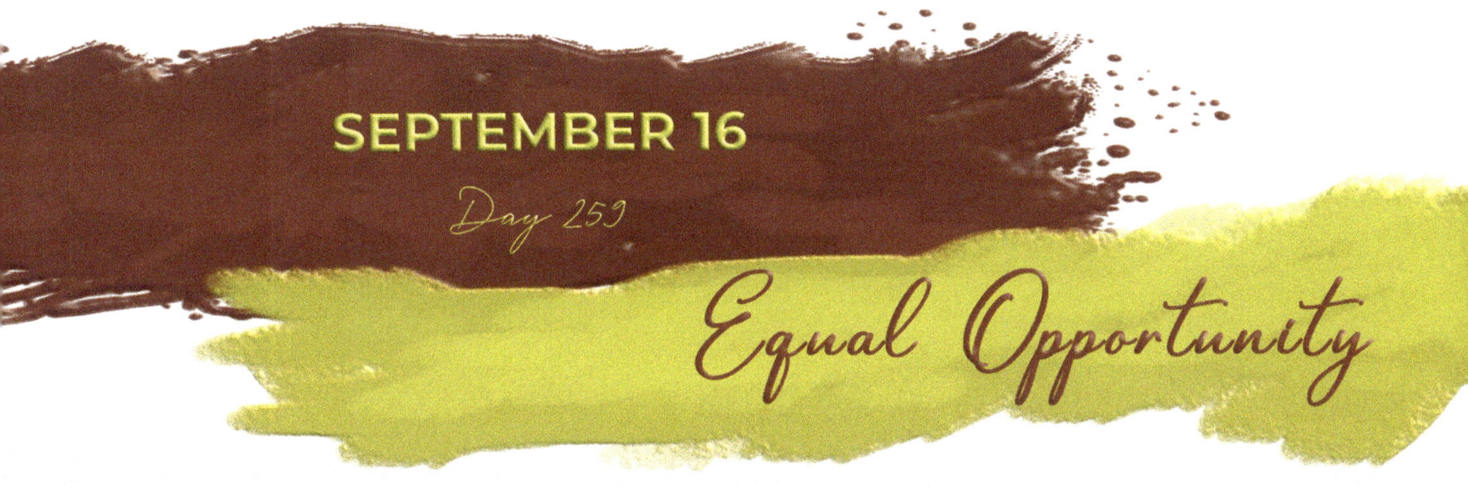

The U.S. Equal Opportunity Employment Commission (EEOC) reviews concerns regarding workplace harassment. The EEOC will investigate complaints and help with a fair resolution. If there is no remedy with your employer, EEOC takes harassment claims seriously, especially involving situations with age, race, sex, color, etc. There are several reasons for workplace burnout, such as heavy workload, untimely deadlines, and weak management. However, a big cause of burnout at work is due to unjust treatment from teammates or supervisors. Unfair treatment may entail bias and favoritism.[273]

Today I will consider equal opportunity in my workplace. Journal about your impressions regarding equal opportunity. Is there anything missing or present about age, race, color, sex, or more, that you notice or have experienced at work? Are there signs of favoritism, bias, or unfair treatment present? How are your workload, deadline timeframe, and management's treatment of employees?

Courtesy of Edward Berkise

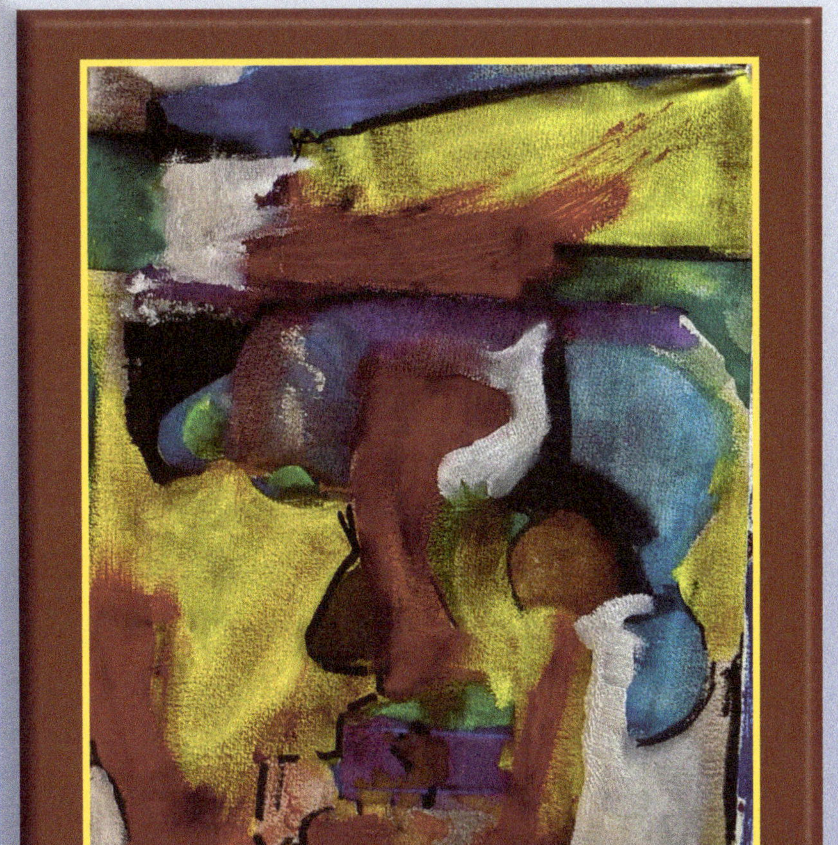

SEPTEMBER 17

Day 260

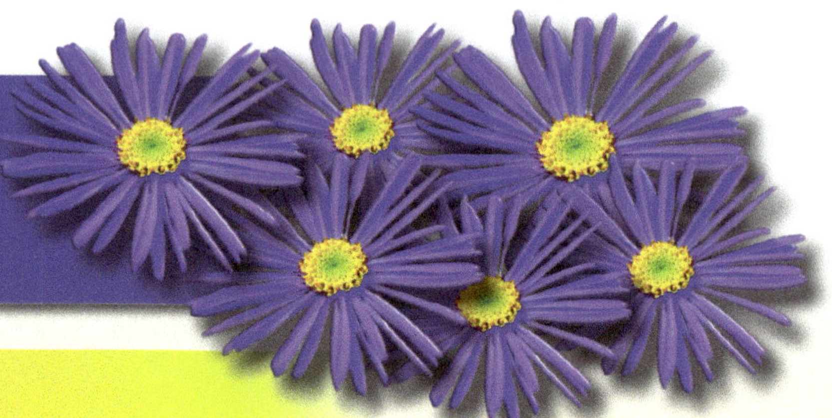

Apologizing

Superfluous expressions of apology for undesirable situations a person is not responsible for are regretful. The apologizer may gain trust by offering a pointless apology. The apologizer attempts to gain trust by demonstrating empathic concern toward the victim. Apologies may have drawbacks, according to some scholars. For instance, repeated superfluous apologies may appear insincere and not yield the expected trust or empathy as a result. On the other hand, even through no fault of their own, an individual can gain trust by merely offering "I'm sorry" for the rain.[274] Are you aware that there is a correct and incorrect way of apologizing? The proper apology is blameless, while an improper apology places blame on another, such as a colleague. The correct way shows your concern without any attached criticism.[275]

Today I will reflect on the way I apologize and the impact it has in the workplace with customers/clients. Do you start sentences with, "I am sorry to bother you?" Consider when you should offer apologies. Journal about a time you had to offer a blameless apology for something in your workplace that kept recurring beyond your control. Did this become exhausting for you? Was it stressful to apologize for something you didn't do? Were you perceived as being sincere? What is your frequency for apologizing for service defects at work?

Courtesy of Jill Santi

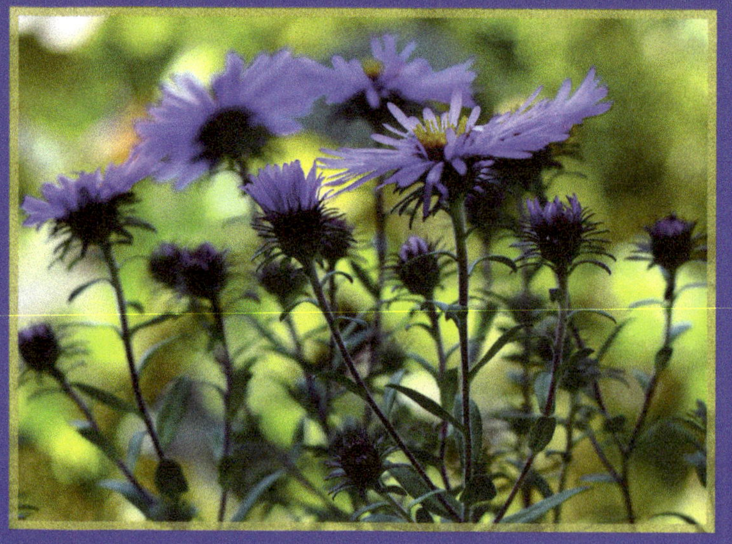

Dancing

Whether you are ballroom dancing, foxtrotting, break dancing, or line dancing – do you realize dancing is very positive for your body and brain? Dancing is incredibly beneficial and has shown positive effects in treating those with neurological movement disorders, such as Parkinson's disease. Music stimulates reward centers in the brain, while dancing activates its motor and sensory circuits. Dance can alleviate stress, increase levels of serotonin (the feel-good hormone), and aid with developing neural connections - particularly in areas involving executive function, spatial recognition, and long-term memory.[276]

Today I will consider the positive effects of dancing. Journal about the last time you remember dancing. Where were you? Who were you with? How did you feel? When was the last time you danced alone in your living room or with your significant other? Dancing reduces stress. With work environments having excessive workloads, short-staffing, documentation demands, and continuous information technology updates, workdays may often cause fatigue. Dancing and music can lift your spirit, offering a form of release.

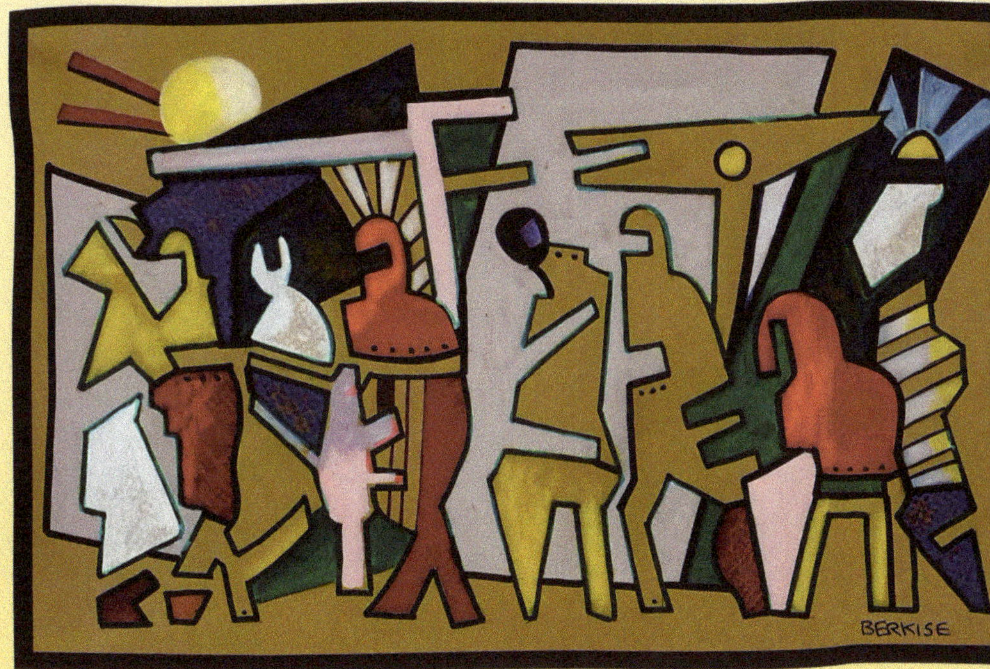

Courtesy of Edward Berkise

SEPTEMBER

19

Day 262

I'm One of a Kind

Remember: I'm one of a kind. Don't forget, if you weren't needed on earth with your unique qualities, you wouldn't have been born. When life is overwhelming you with problems and challenges, a single person can make all the difference. Actually, it is one person that changes the things that matter. Strive to be that person.[277]

Today I will realize I am one of a kind. Journal about whether you are one to "buck the system" or whether you "go with the flow." In order to be one of a kind, you must not be afraid to be yourself. When you are your authentic self, that is when you are most creative. This is what companies need most to be a success! Over time, work cultures have become homogeneous, often resulting in group thinking and inadvertently omitting cognitive diversity. Expressing yourself as "one of a kind" may be a challenge to your authentic self as well as the organization you work for. This flux can be stressful and create moral distress. How will you make a difference in the world today?

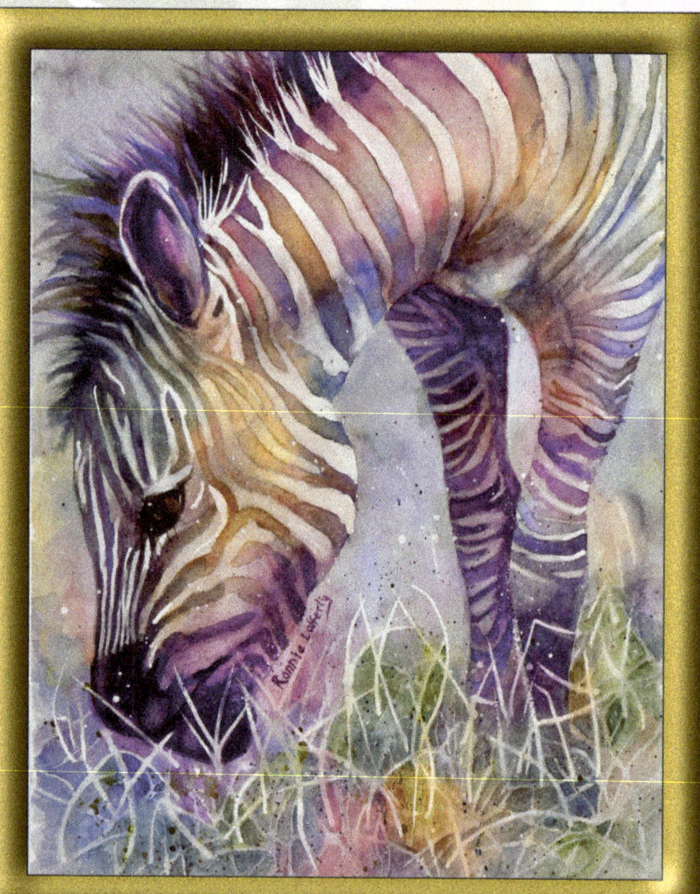

Courtesy of Ronnie Lafferty

SEPTEMBER 20

Day 263

Living Joy

Living joy involves passion, inspiration, and motivation. It's about creating goals while taking time to do things that make you happy. Experiencing living joy benefits your entire body, especially your mind and heart. Research suggests joyful people may have a smaller risk of having a cardiac event, maintaining healthy cholesterol, better blood pressure, optimal weight, and decreased stress. Studies also show that joyful people are likelier to eat healthier foods, exercise more, sleep well, and refrain from smoking. Living joy brings you better wellness and health.[278]

Today I will rate my level of joy, with 10 being the highest and 1 being the lowest. If you are 8 and above, that's pretty good. If you are 5 to 8, you have some opportunity to increase your joy. If you are 1-5, you may feel miserable and need to evaluate what you are doing with your life and what is missing. Consider seeking mental health support. Journal about your joy level and think of three things you can do to bring more happiness into your life. Make your plans for living joy.

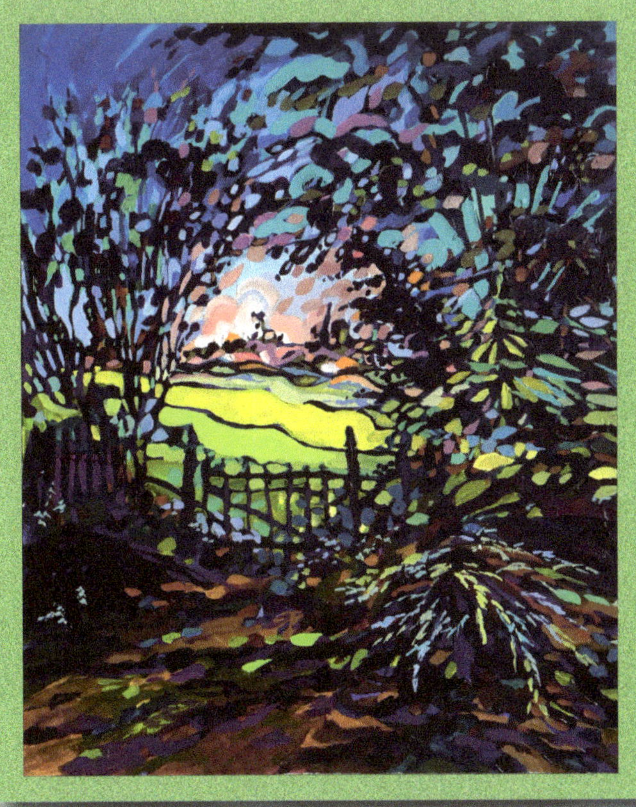

Courtesy of Judy Hodge

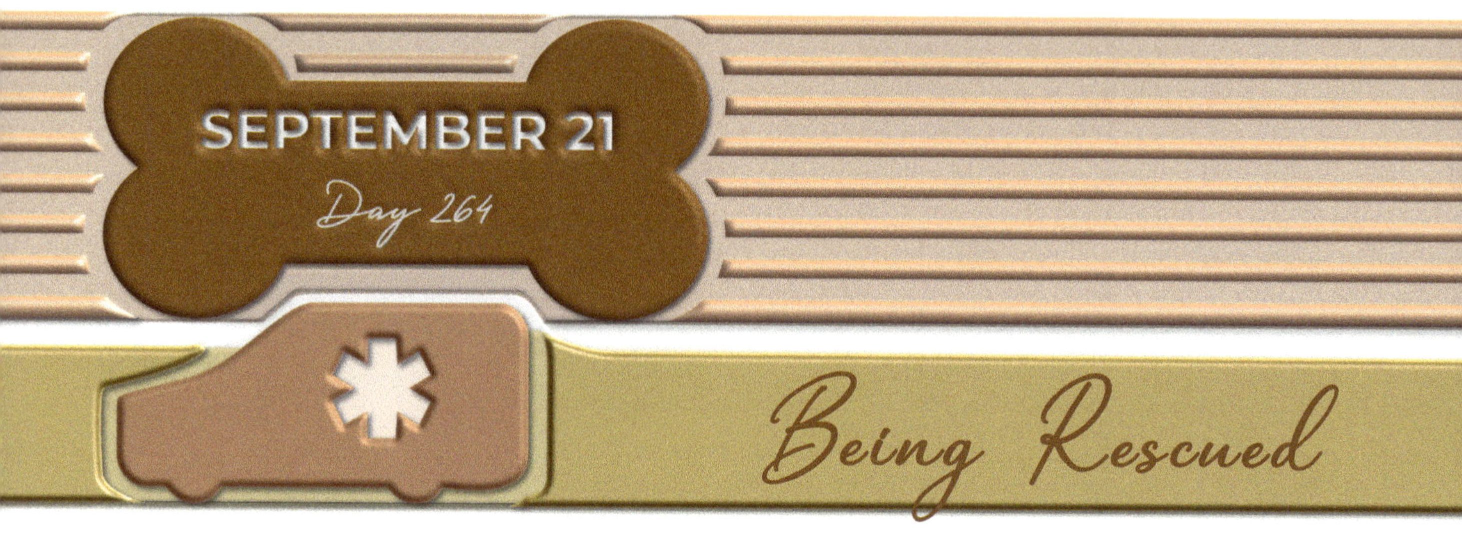

SEPTEMBER 21

Day 264

Being Rescued

The Underground Railroad had confidential routes and safe houses in the U.S. during the earlier to mid-1800s. African American slaves took these routes, escaping to Canada or free states with the help of allies and abolitionists sympathetic to the cause. The Underground Railroad sympathizers infiltrated and acted to rescue oppressed people. Today, we must fight against modern-day slavery. Similar parallels exist between "historic versus modern-day sex trafficking slavery of minors and adults."[279]

Today I will remember if I ever needed to be rescued. Journal about what the circumstances were. Think about historical and modern-day slaves in distress, the need to be rescued, and how peoples' lives may parallel situations in the past. Do you know someone who may need rescuing? Learn more about the National Human Trafficking Hotline at 1 (888-373-7888).[280] Improving social awareness of others around you that may be in need of rescuing is critical due to rising estimates of hundreds of thousands of trafficking victims in the U.S., Mexico, and the Philippines.

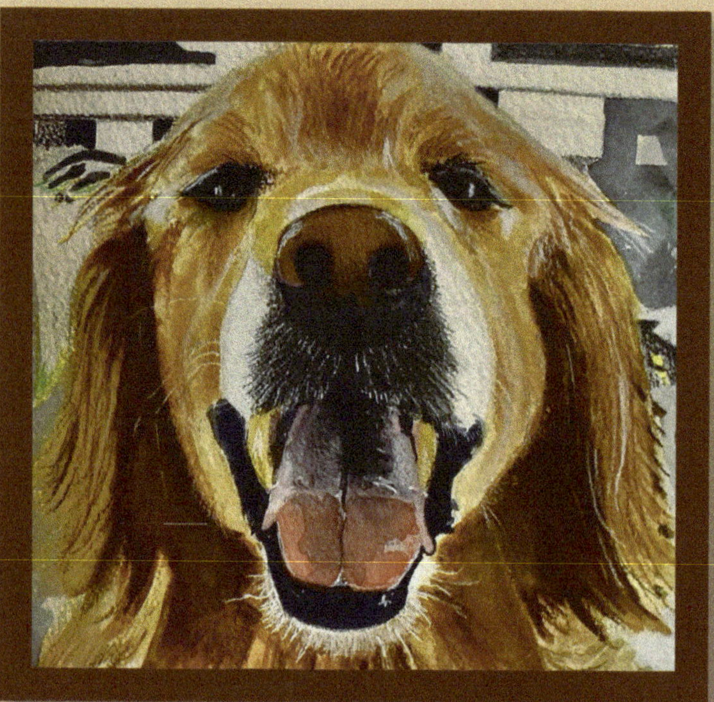

Courtesy of Edward Berkise

Shaping the Future

Forces of technology and globalization are changing our workplaces, economies, families, and communities. In emerging and advanced economies, job disruption, decelerating growth, a broken social contract, and rising inequality create instability. However, this is the best time for mobilizing technology and for unleashing the human potential for addressing these problems to shape an improved socioeconomic system that offers opportunities for everyone.[281]

Today I will consider how our future is being shaped. Journal about any disruptions, instabilities, or stagnant growth you may have experienced recently, especially with the Covid-19 pandemic. What things do you expect to change as a result of the effects of Covid-19 with healthcare, in the workplace, your home life, and public gatherings? How will you navigate the future with social distancing as the new reality? How will you shape your future with the increased potential for being isolated?

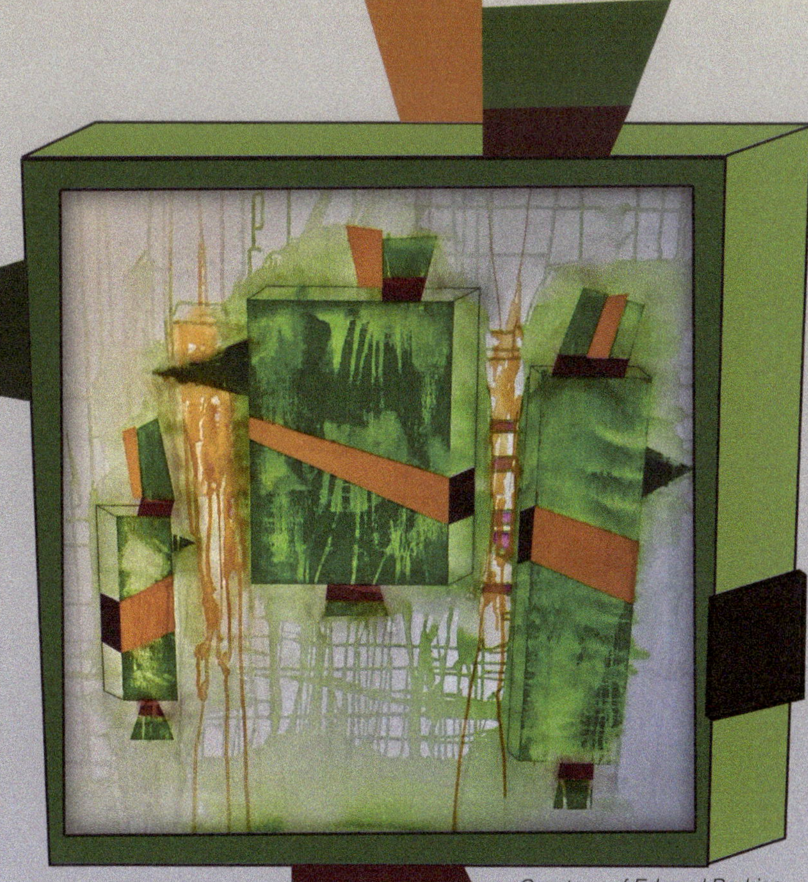

Courtesy of Edward Berkise

SEPTEMBER 23

Day 266

Go Further than Before

What is in your backpack? Sometimes carrying extra things needlessly creates clutter, even metaphorically, such as tumultuous relationships, unhealthy habits, or thoughts that do not serve us. Perhaps the clutter creates false narratives in our mind that makes us feel secure. Truthfully, the over cluttered backpack is not sustainable for leading an independent, above-average lifestyle. Those extra items in your backpack keep you from living a life of efficiency. They also prevent pursuing and obtaining your dreams. What can you let go of to create the life you imagine? What keeps you from success? Do you seek familiarity and comfort, or passion and adventure? Remove unnecessary items from your backpack. Keep unique skills, needed tools, and only essential things for survival. Look to the path ahead, the route you are yearning to take. There are amazing opportunities if you allow yourself to go further than before.[282]

Today I will consider the things that hold me back. Journal about everything holding you back from reaching or making a new goal for yourself. List out specifics. Making lists that you can see helps make you more self-aware of the things you need to accomplish. Checking those things off your list or putting a line through them when you have finished the task creates a feeling of actualization and self-pride.

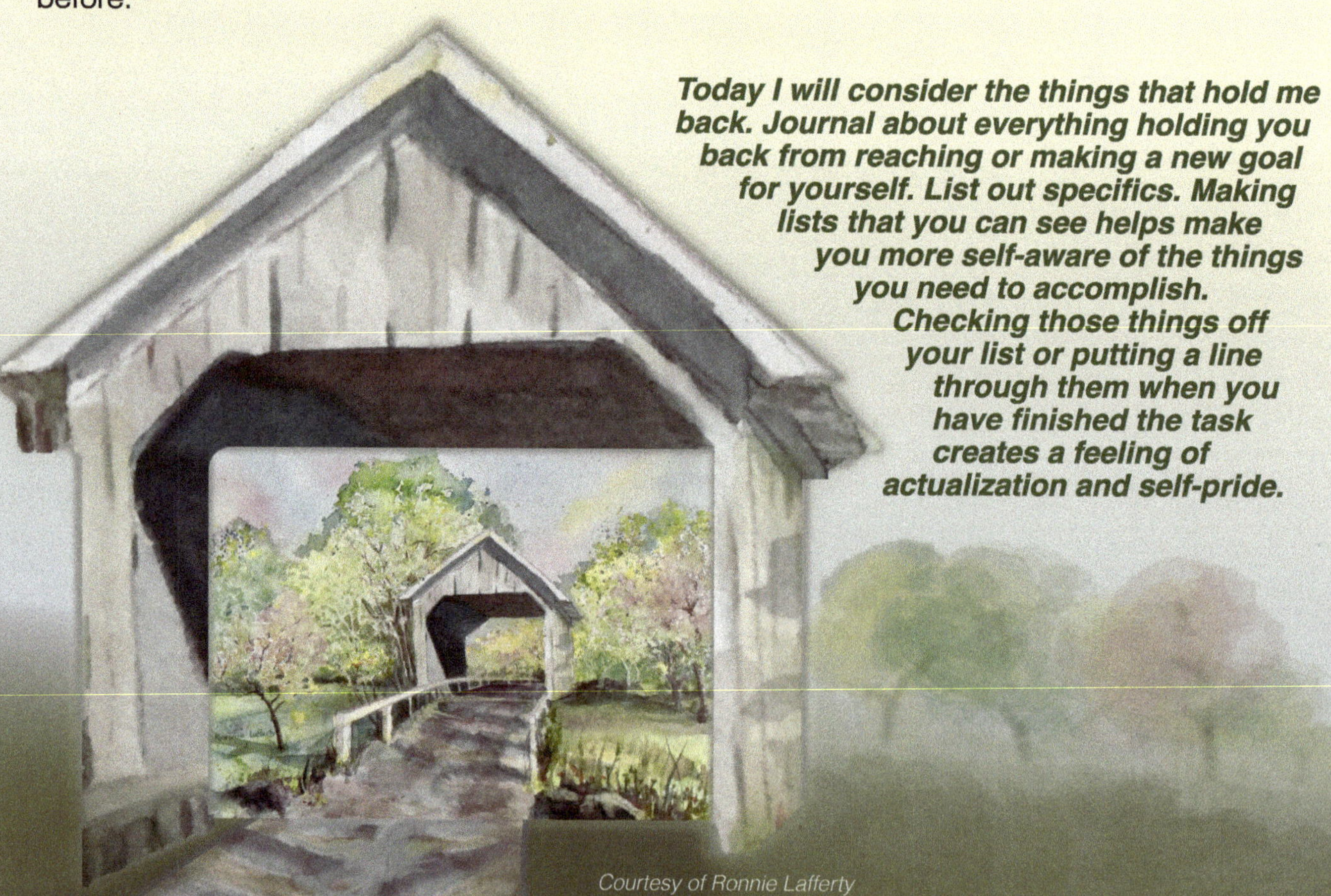

Courtesy of Ronnie Lafferty

SEPTERMBER 24

Day 267

Forgiving

It is simpler to say you forgive than to do it. Many people feel that forgiveness means approving an incident. However, it is not. Blame binds us to our past and diminishes the size of our heart and mind—both metaphorically and literally. However, forgiving means we realize that hatred and resentment cause more pain. Science proves that forgiving is beneficial to your health. Forgiveness does not mean that you forget. It's not justifying, accepting, or overlooking any occurrences, either. It's simply making the choice to let go of your resentment or feelings of wanting revenge. Through forgiving, we are eliminating our suffering, not the misconduct. The offender may not deserve to be pardoned, but you merit feeling at peace. When forgiving, you are setting yourself free.[283]

Today I will think about whom I have not forgiven. When you don't forgive, it harms you, not the other person. Not forgiving causes stress, disharmony, sometimes physiological aches and pains, fomented anger, and eventual exhaustion. This contributes to poor focus if unable to separate the unrelenting ruminations from the job at hand. Sometimes it takes a little time to forgive, and that's okay. Journal about the possibility of forgiving that person today, not for them, but for you and your wellbeing.

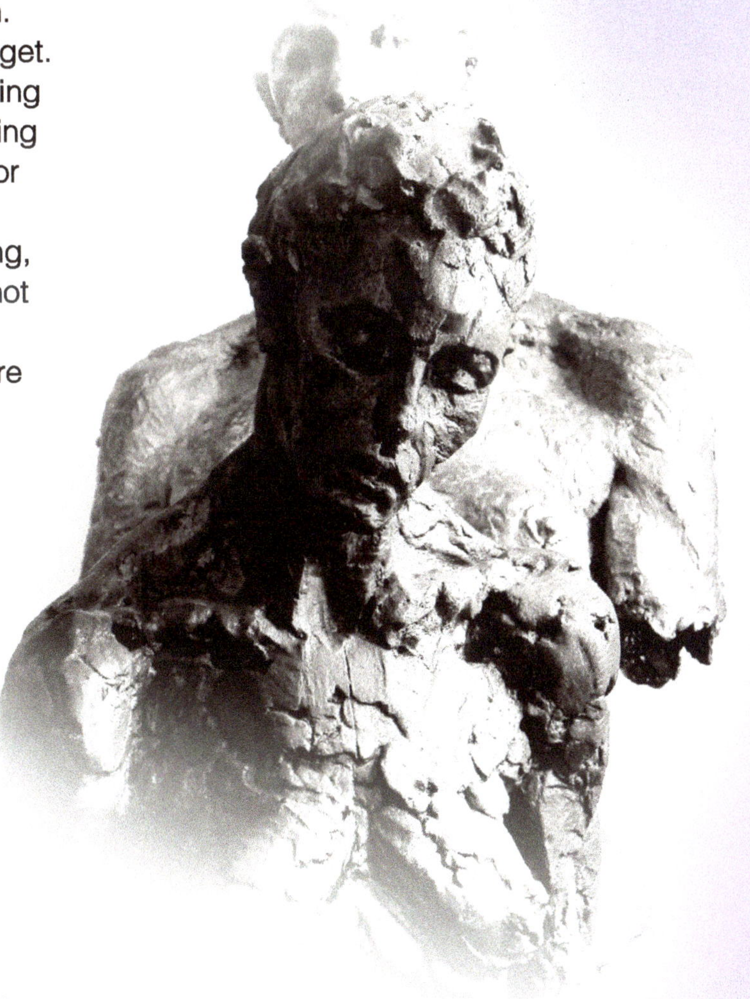

Courtesy of Umberto Kamperveen

Actualizing

There's a difference between basic needs and growth needs, according to Maslow. Needs occurring under self-actualization in Maslow's pyramid are basic needs. When basic needs are not satisfied, it creates the feeling that something is void from our lives, which leads to feelings of tension and exhibiting neurotic behaviors. For instance, not having a roof over our heads threatens our sense of security. This problem will completely dominate our being until we meet our basic needs. Once these needs are met, we can then move toward focusing on our growth needs. Basic needs are external, whereas needs related to growth are internal. Growth needs motivate us from deep within ourselves, and we no longer depend on other's thoughts, such as friends, family, and coworkers.[284]

Today I will consider actualizing and my basic needs. Are you presently actualizing? Are your basic needs being met? Journal about your basic needs and outline your growth needs. How do you envision moving beyond your basic needs to your growth needs? What steps can you take now? When we don't actualize our needs, it's frustrating and may lead to cynicism and/or moral distress.

Courtesy of Ann Parker

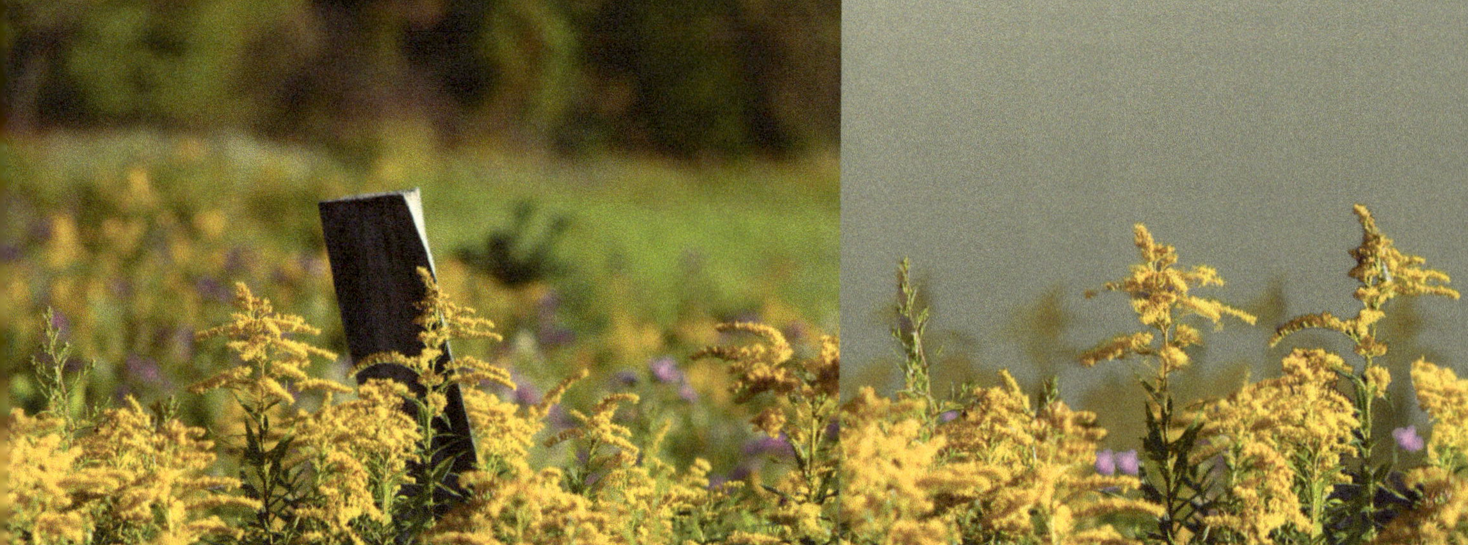

SEPTEMBER 26

Day 269

The Bigger Picture

Do you go into your kitchen and see only dirty dishes? Open your kitchen cabinets and take notice of just how many dishes are clean. I laughed out loud after trying this. I never really focused on the clean things in my kitchen. When doing so, things didn't seem so bad. Acknowledging the clean dishes in our kitchen cabinets allows us to see the bigger picture. We stop focusing so much on what perturbs us and expand the whole vista within our life. Stop looking for faults and pay attention to what is glorious and wonderful. This goes further than pessimism or optimism. See life entirely and acknowledge everything. In fact, there are many thanks to give. See the bigger picture and realize just how much is really going your way.[285]

Today I will "open my kitchen cabinets" and consider all that is going well for me today. Journal about the bigger picture and reflect on all the beautiful things happening in your life that bring you joy rather than stress, anger, exhaustion, and other negative feelings. Practice being thankful at work, not just at home. Can you see the entire vista of your life? Do you see dirty or clean dishes in your kitchen?

Courtesy of Edward Berkise

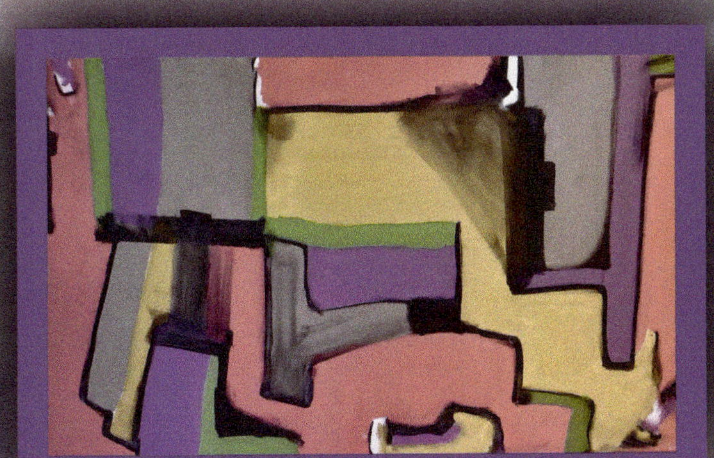

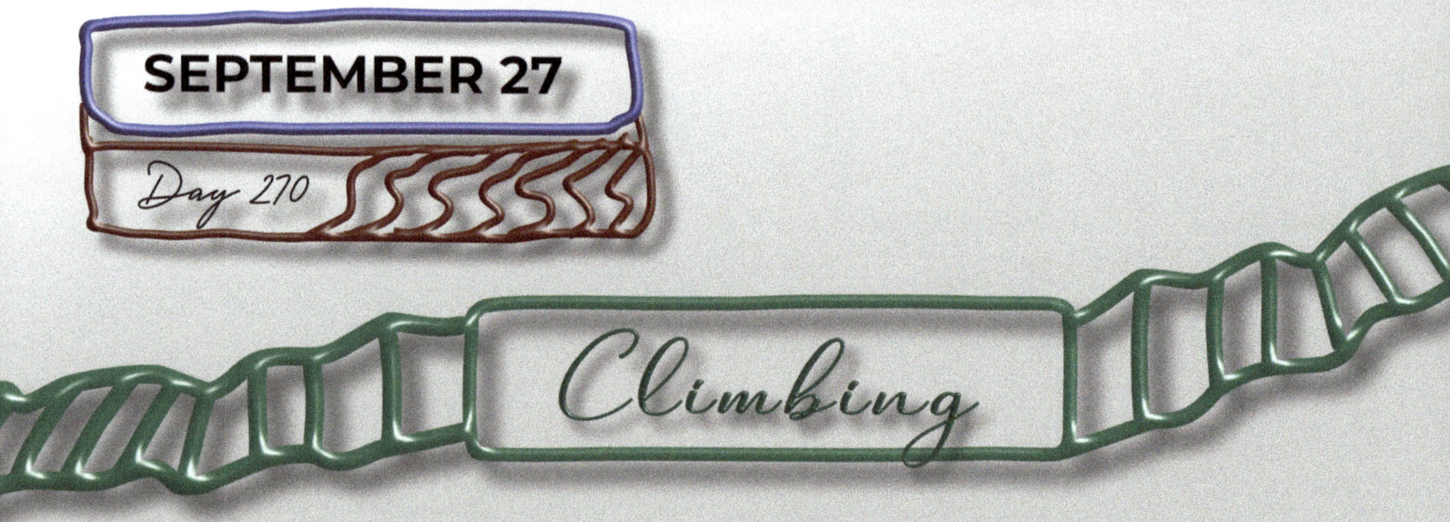

Climbing is often hard, but it can also be the most gratifying accomplishment. Climbing takes us places with amazing beauty and challenges us to tap into our reserves of resourcefulness and strength. It can also be a lot of fun if you are willing to put in some effort. For many of us, it is our life work, while others see it as a detour on their way to better things. However, climbing becomes a devotion, which naturally comes to us all.[286] Conventional wisdom tells us the path to success is staying in your own lane, meeting others within your industry, and climbing the corporate ladder. Research suggests that when you develop a tight-knit group of contacts from a single industry or work on a single path, it is far less valuable than building a network that spans groups and industries.[287]

Today I will consider that not every generation wants to climb the ladder or mountain. For instance, the millennials want fast results, and sticking to a traditional 8-5 job isn't what they have in mind. If they get bored, millennials may just start up a new, brighter, and bolder company rather than follow the older generations with corporate ladder climbing mindsets.[288] Journal about how you go about climbing, and if you think or feel your method is effective. Tap into resourcefulness and strength reserves should you choose to climb.

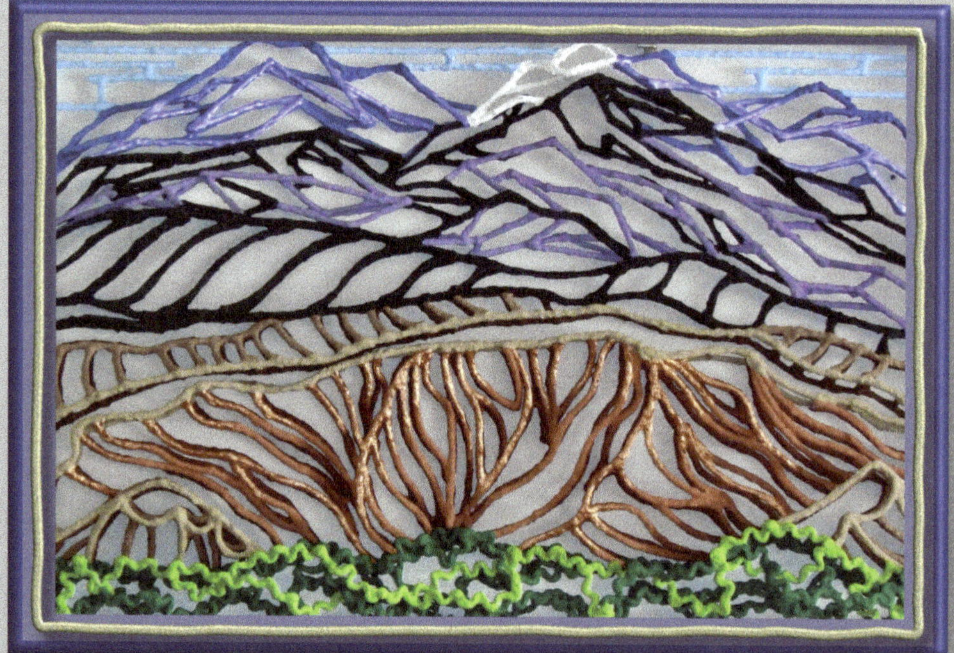

Courtesy of Jon Chisholm

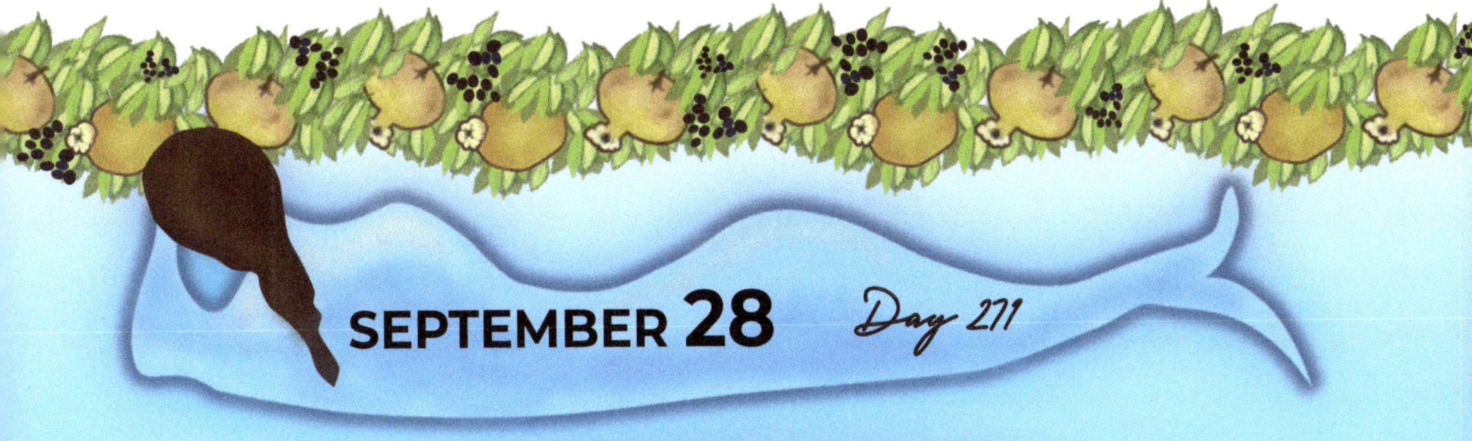

Having Some Fun

You must realize that things you find fun may not be fun for someone else. Fun is often difficult to evaluate using standard scientific methods. Scientific conclusions regarding the benefits of fun derive from "subjective observations and less rigorous studies." There are plenty of studies indirectly connecting to concepts of fun and play - there is a case for us needing more fun.[289]

Today, besides work projects, I will consider what other things I do for fun. Life isn't meant to be about working all the time. You need hobbies, self-care activities, and enjoy some fun. Journal about the things you like to do for fun. How much fun have you had today, this week, month, or year? Do you put off having fun, or do you make it a priority like your work? What is the last thing you did that was fun?

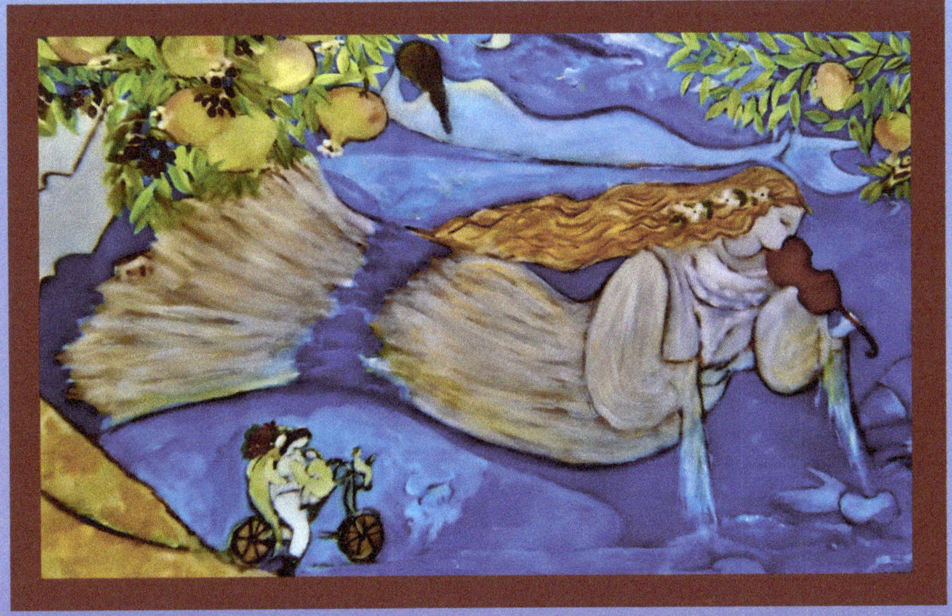

Courtesy of Maika Gonzalez

SEPTEMBER 29

Day 272

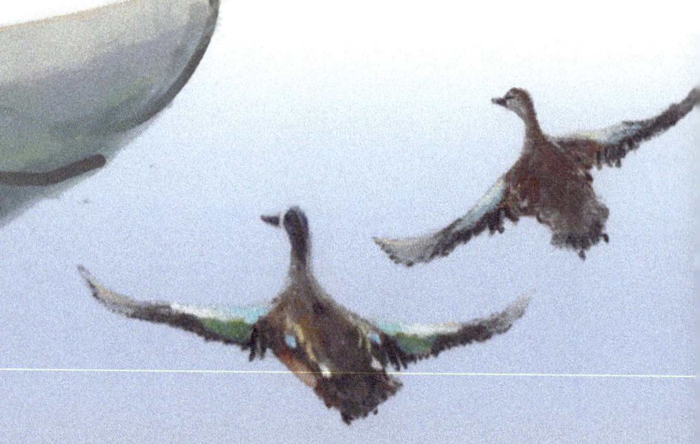

Meaningful Connections

Our society has become technology-obsessed. We may have more friends on Facebook than we do in person. We can easily hide behind our computer screens, comfortable at home scrolling, swiping, and texting. This can make it a real challenge to make a rewarding connection.[290] In our social media age, it is so important to make genuine connections. It's tempting to eye-roll when folks say they are friends with certain people and later discover they may only be connected through social media. They never met in person or actually communicated with them, yet they call them friends.[291]

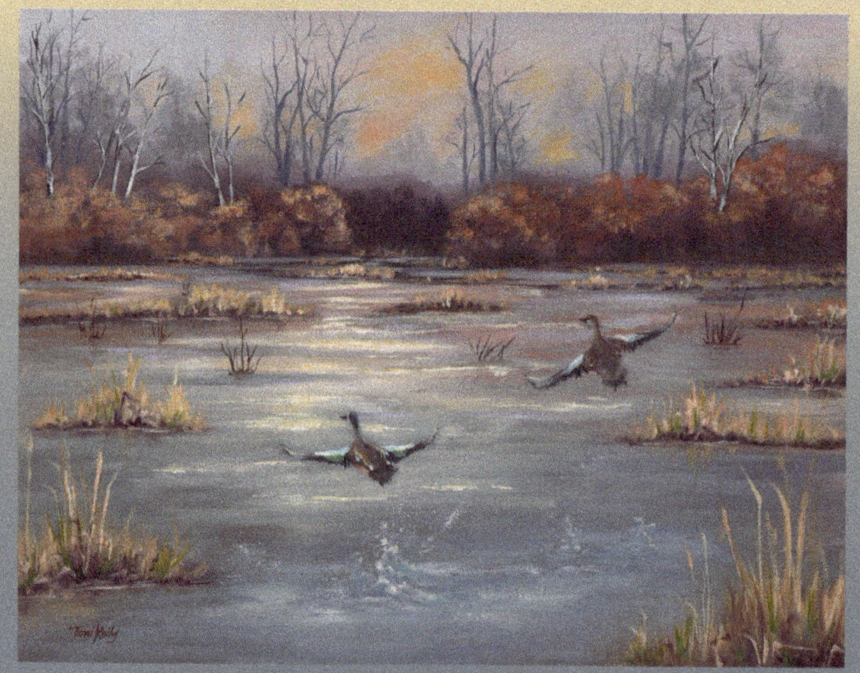

Courtesy of Toni Kelly

Today I will consider my meaningful relationships and make deliberate connections. Describe in your journal how you go about making rewarding connections. Whether at work or home, the meaningful connections you make offer support when you feel stressed or need to talk with someone. Evaluate if your connections are genuine.

SEPTEMBER 30

Day 273

Don't Lie to Me

"It is true that truth lives and lies die. It is true that an honest man finally triumphs, but it is the temporary period of harm that comes to the honest man that we are trying to point out. You can tell five people a lie about a certain man, and the gossipers will spread the news and make the innocent man suffer greatly until the lie is killed by the truth coming out. There are two kinds of liars; the unthinking, and the malicious liar. One lies without a purpose and the other with a purpose - both are bad, but the latter especially so."[292] Lies are damaging to democratic processes. Blatantly incorrect political statements about policy aim at the core of democracy. If both sides never agree on facts, then making judgments about government or accountability is impossible.[293]

Today I will consider the damage caused by lying. Did your parents teach you as a child that you shouldn't lie? Lies are harmful and can lead to burnout.[294] Write in your journal the earliest memories you have about being taught not to lie. Who discussed this with you? Was it your parents, pastor, siblings, or friends? Lies are often childish, malicious, or unthinking, and temporary until truth prevails. Sometimes people tell little white lies. However, people may lie because they have an agenda.

Courtesy of Marla Julien

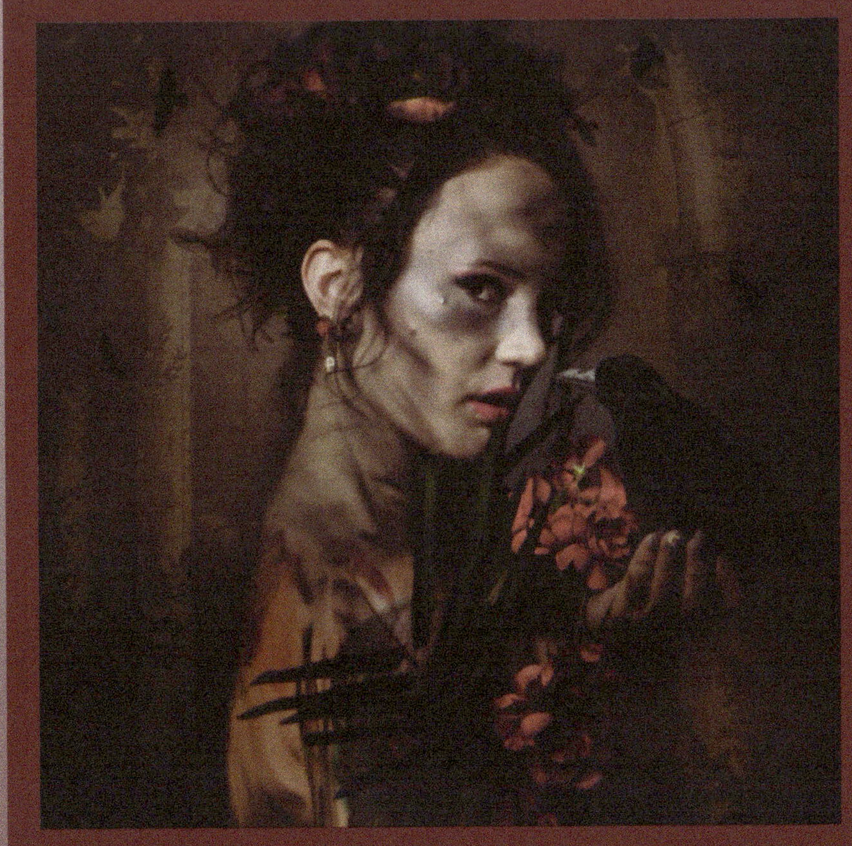

References

[1]National Academy of Sciences. Taking Action Against Clinician Burnout: A Systems Approach to Professional Well-Being. National Academy of Medicine. Consensus Study Report. 2019 Oct. https://nam.edu/wp-content/uploads/2019/10/CR-report-hightlights-brief-final.pdf.. Accessed December 9, 2019.

[2]AMN Leadership Solutions. 2020 Healthcare Trends. AMN Healthcare. 2020. https://www.amnhealthcare.com/uploadedFiles/MainSite/Content/Campaigns/10-healthcare-trends-white-paper-2020.pdf.. Accessed April 14, 2020.

[3]National Academy of Sciences. Taking Action Against Clinician Burnout: A Systems Approach to Professional Well-Being. National Academy of Medicine. Consensus Study Report. 2019 Oct. https://nam.edu/wp-content/uploads/2019/10/CR-report-hightlights-brief-final.pdf.. Accessed December 9, 2019.

[194]Penfold J, Collier J. Physicians: Five Extraordinary Hobbies to Keep Burnout at Bay. Medical News Today. 2018 Jan. https://www.medicalnewstoday.com/articles/320526. Accessed February 26, 2020.

[195]Pillars W. Six Signs of -and Solutions for- Teacher Burnout. Education Week Teacher. 2014 May. https://www.edweek.org/tm/articles/2014/05/20/ctq-pillars-signs-of-solutions-for-burnout.html. Accessed March 1, 2020.

[196]King J. 3 Reasons 'Practice Makes Perfect'. SMART Recovery. 2018 Jan. https://www.smart recovery.org/3-reasons-practice-makes-perfect/. Accessed March 4, 2020.

[197]Mirpuri M. What Does Independence Mean to Me? Maheka Mirpuri. 2016 Jan. https://maheka mirpuri.com/what-does-independence-mean-to-me/. Accessed March 4, 2020.

[198]Swoboda K. Not Getting What You Want? Good! Your Courageous Life. 2019 Jan. https://www.yourcourageouslife.com/not-getting-what-you-want-good/. Accessed March 4, 2020.

[199]Jones JE. The Power of the Olive Branch. The Inspiration Report: Beliefnet. 2011 Apr. https://www.beliefnet.com/columnists/inspirationreport/2011/04/the-power-of-the-olive-branch.html. Accessed March 4, 2020.

[200]Half R. How to Get the Recognition at Work you Deserve. Robert Half: Job Seeker. 2016 Apr. https://www.roberthalf.com/blog/salaries-and-skills/how-to-get-the-recognition-at-work-you- deserve. Accessed February 1, 2020.

[201]VIA Institute on Character. Prudence: Become Aware of 2Your Strength. VIA Institute. 2020. https://www.viacharacter.org/character-strengths/prudence. Accessed March 6, 2020.

[202]Jiang L, Probst T. If You Live in an Area with High Income Inequality, You're More Likely to Burn Out at Work. Harvard Business Review. 2017 July. https://hbr.org/2017/05/if-you- live-in-an-area-with-high-income-inequality-youre-more-likely-to-burn-out-at-work. Accessed March 8, 2020.

[203]A Place at Home- Omaha. Caregivers: Making an Impact Isn't Always Easy. NE0001. 2019 Oct. https://www.aplaceathome.com/ne0001/news/caregiverimpact/. Accessed March 6, 2020.

[204]Schwartz T. Why Appreciation Matters So Much. Harvard Business Review. 2012 Jan. https://hbr.org/2012/01/why-appreciation-matters-so-mu. Accessed March 8, 2020.

[205]Shaheen S. Don't Stress Me Out! The News International: Latest News Breaking, Pakistan News. 2016 Mar. https://www.thenews.com.pk/magazine/you/101802-dont-stress-me-out. Accessed March 8, 2020.

[206]Juma N. 105 Awesome Quotes on Knowing Your Worth and Value. Everyday Power. 2020 Feb. https://everydaypower.com/know-your-worth-quotes/. Accessed March 8, 2020.

[207]Workingamerica.org. Not Being Paid Fairly. Working America. 0AD. https://www.working america.org/fixmyjob/compensation//not-being-paid-fairly. Accessed March 8, 2020.

[208]Zalis S. Our Stories Matter: Use Your Voice to Share Your Workplace Lessons. Forbes. 2018 Jan. https://www.forbes.com/sites/shelleyzalis/2018/01/18/find-your-voice-share-your- story/#f1d9a071a2ee. Accessed March 6, 2018.

[209]Knaus B. Protect Yourself from Pushy People. Psychology Today. 2012 Mar. https://www.psychologytoday.com/us/blog/science-and-sensibility/201203/protect-yourself-pushy-people. Accessed March 8, 2020.

[210]Washington K. Balancing Work, Life, and Caregiving: You Can't Go it Alone AgingCare. 2017 Aug. https://www.agingcare.com/articles/balancing-career-caregiving-cant-do-it-alone- 180295.htm. Accessed March 9, 2020.

[211]Freed J. Why We Overcommit & How to Stop. Goop. 2018 Dec. https://goop.com/wellness/ mindfulness/why-we-overcommit/. Accessed March 10, 2020.

[212]Bocco D. 10 Ways to Pursue Happiness. HowStuffWorks. 2020 Jan. https://science.howstuff works.com/life/inside-the-mind/emotions/10-ways-pursue-happiness3.htm. Accessed March 10, 2020.

[213]Khan MN. What is Classed as Gross Misconduct in the Workplace? Truth Legal Solicitors. 2019 June. https://www.truthlegal.com/what-is-classed-as-gross-misconduct-in-the-workplace/. Accessed March 10, 2020.

[214]McSorley E. Breaking Up Workplace Cliques. The Predictive Index. 2016 Dec. https://www. predictiveindex.com/blog/breaking-up-workplace-cliques/. Accessed March 10, 2020.

[215]Jacobs D. How Can I be Relevant and Important to People? Quora. 2015 Nov. https://www.quora.com/How-can-I-be-relevant-and-important-to-people. Accessed March 10, 2020.

[216]Whitmore J. 7 Ways to Create Harmony in the Office. Entrepreneur. 2016 Apr. https://www.entrepreneur.com/article/274367. Accessed March 10, 2020.

[217]Belli G. How to Set Better Boundaries at Work. PayScale. 2019 Apr. https://www.payscale. com/career-news/2019/04/how-to-set-better-boundaries-at-work. Accessed March 10, 2020.

[218]Cunha D. Childcare and Working Parents: The Juggle is Real. Explore Parents. 2019. https://www.parents.com/parenting/work/stay-home/childcare-and-working-parents-the- juggle-is-real/. Accessed March 26, 2020.

[219]Moss D. 5 Generations + 7 Values = Endless Opportunities. SHRM. 2017 June. https://www. shrm.org/hr-today/news/hr-news/conference-today/pages/2017/5-generations-7-values- endless-opportunities.aspx. Accessed March 26, 2020.

[220]Mowry T. The Benefits of Taking Time Off. Tamera Mowry. 2014 Sep. http://www.tamera mowry.com/time-benefits-taking-time/. Accessed March 26, 2020.

[221]Cho J. 6 Scientifically Proven Benefits of Mindfulness and Meditation. Forbes. 2016 July. https://www.forbes.com/sites/jeenacho/2016/07/14/10-scientifically-proven-benefits-of-mindfulness-and-meditation/#288b781863ce. Accessed March 26, 2020.

[222]Augustin S. Looking Out The Window, What Should You See? Psychology Today. 2018 Mar. https://www.psychologytoday.com/us/blog/people-places-and-things/201803/looking-out-the- window-what-should-you-see. Accessed March 26, 2020.

[223]Therapist Aid. What are Personal Boundaries? UHS Berkeley. 2016. https://uhs.berkeley.edu/ sites/default/files/relationships_personal_boundaries.pdf. Accessed March 26, 2020.

[224]Muller R. Why Work Gossip is Bad for You, and How to Stop Doing It. Thrive Global. 2019 June. https://thriveglobal.com/stories/work-gossip-stress-levels-toxic-environment-how-to- avoid/. Accessed March 27, 2020.

[225]Hunter WC. No Need to Despair. Think a Book for Today. Chicago, IL: The Reilly & Britton Company; (1918):9, 33.

[226]Thaik C. Self-Doubt Destroys the Heart, Mind, Body and Soul. HuffPost. 2013 June. https://www.huffpost.com/entry/self-doubt_b_2960936. Accessed March 27, 2020.

[227]Clear J. Grit: A Complete Guide on How to Be More Mentally Tough. James Clear. 0AD. https://jamesclear.com/grit. Accessed March 27, 2020.

[228]Løvseth LT, Aasland OG, Fridner A, et al. Confidentiality as a Barrier to Support Seeking Among Physicians: The Influence of Psychological Work Factors in Four European Hospitals (The HOUPE Study). PubMed. Work. 2014;49(1):113-121. https://pubmed.ncbi.nlm.nih. gov/24004783/. Accessed March 27, 2020.

[229]Joshi B. Being the Good Guy at Work is a Bad Idea. Entrepreneur. 2018 Oct. https://www.entrepreneur.com/article/321793. Accessed April 12, 2020.

[230]SMART Goal – Definition, Guide, and Importance of Goal Setting. Corporate Finance Institute. 2020. https://corporatefinanceinstitute.com/resources/knowledge/other/smart-goal/. Accessed April 12, 2020.

[231]Fadel L. In These Divided Times, Is Civility Under Siege? NPR. 2019 Mar. https://www.npr. org/2019/03/12/702011061/in-these-divided-times-is-civility-under-siege. Accessed April 12, 2020.

[232]Tsdf. What is Social Justice? The San Diego Foundation. 2016 Mar. https://www.sd foundation.org/news-events/sdf-news/what-is-social-justice/. Accessed April 12, 2020.

[233]Carrisi CBP, SP. Own Your Mistakes: Cristel Carrisi at TEDxZagreg (Transcript). The Singju Post. 2020 Jan. https://singjupost.com/own-your-mistakes-cristel-carrisi-at-tedxzagreb- transcript/. Accessed April 13, 2020.

[234]Holly K. Dealing with Verbal Abuse at Work. HealthyPlace. 2020. https://www.healthyplace. com/abuse/verbal-abuse/dealing-with-verbal-abuse-at-work. Accessed April 14, 2020.

[235]Make-A-Wish America. 2020. https://wish.org/. Accessed April 14, 2020.

[236]Johnson JA. The Psychology of Expectations. Psychology Today. 2018 Feb. https://www.psychologytoday.com/us/blog/cui-bono/201802/the-psychology-expectations. Accessed April 15, 2020.

[237]Mayhew R. Does Getting Terminated from a Job Make it Harder to Find Another Job? Chron. 2018 June. https://work.chron.com/getting-terminated-job-make-harder-another-job- 22460.html. Accessed April 15, 2020.

[238]The Rutten Law Firm, APC. My Boss is a Jerk! Can I Sue Him? The Rutten Law Firm: Employment Law Opportunities. 2013 Feb. https://www.californialegaladvocates.com/blog/2013/02/my-boss-is-a-jerk-can-i-sue-him.shtml. Accessed April 15, 2020.

[239]Shelton T. Everybody Isn't your Friend. AZ Quotes. 2013 Nov. https://www.azquotes.com/quote/820858?ref=got-your-back. Accessed April 15, 2020.

[240]Alton L. 7 Practical Tips to Achieve a Positive Mindset. SUCCESS. 2019 June. https://www. success.com/7-practical-tips-to-achieve-a-positive-mindset/. Accessed April 15, 2020.

[241]Perera C. 23 Scientific Ways to be Popular at Work. CreditDonkey. 2019 May. https://www.creditdonkey.com/popular-work.html. Accessed April 15, 2020.

[242]Shiao V. Drawing the Line with Work Friends. The Business Times. 2018 Aug. https://www. businesstimes.com.sg/opinion/cubicle-files/drawing-the-line-with-work-friends. Accessed April 15, 2020.

[243]Webb L. How to be a Nimble Thinker. Training Journal. 2016 Feb. https://www.training journal.com/articles/feature/how-be-nimble-thinker. Accessed April 15, 2020.

[244]Ferro G. Human Resources is Not Your Friend. EtherealMind. 2017 July. https://etherealmind. com/human-resources-is-not-your-friend/. Accessed April 15, 2020.

[245]Kramer B. Council Post: Why It's Time to Stop Labeling Ourselves and Those Around Us. Forbes. 2019 May. https://www.forbes.com/sites/forbescoachescouncil/2019/05/21/why-its- time-to-stop-labeling-ourselves-and-those-around-us/#2e5b2a3e433d. Accessed April 15, 2020.

[246]Hubbard E. Elbert Hubbard Quotes. Brainy Quote. 1918. https://www.brainyquote.com/quotes/elbert_hubbard_106845. Accessed April 15, 2020.

[247]Seieg C. Could You Get PTSD From Your Pandemic Experience? The Long-Term Mental Health Effects of Coronavirus. CNBC. 2020 Apr. https://www.cnbc.com/2020/04/17/long- term-mental-health-ptsd-effects-of-covid-19-pandemic-explained.html. Accessed April 19, 2020.

[248]Workopolis. How to Get a Job Without Experience (When No One Will Hire You Without Experience). Workopolis Blog. 2015 Sep. https://careers.workopolis.com/advice/how-to-get- a-job-without-any-experience-when-no-one-will-hire-you-without-experience/. Accessed April 19, 2020.

[249]Webb M. 5 Ways to Ensure Your Judgment is Sound. Forbes. 2016 Oct. https://www.forbes. com/sites/maynardwebb/2016/10/24/the-good-and-the-bad-on-judgment/#489e918578d0. Accessed April 19, 2020.

[250]Onley D. Georgia Nurse Who Quit Over COVID-19 Has Second Thoughts. TheGrio. 2020 Apr. https://thegrio.com/2020/04/02/georgia-nurse-covid-19/. Accessed April 19, 2020.

[251]Hornigold T. We're Making Progress in Explainable AI, but Major Pitfalls Remain. Singularity Hub. 2019 Nov. https://singularityhub.com/2019/11/18/the-progress-were-making-in-explainable-ai-and-the-pitfalls-that-remain/. Accessed April 19, 2020.

[252]Healthwise Staff. Stress Management: Relaxing your Mind and Body. CS Mott Children's Hospital – Michigan Medicine. 2016 Mar. https://www.mottchildren.org/health- library/uz2209. Accessed April 19, 2020.

[253]Masterson L, May W, Karnopp W, et al. The Critical Inner Voice Explained. PsychAlive. 2018 Apr. https://www.psychalive.org/critical-inner-voice/. Accessed April 20, 2020.

[254]Lipsy L. How to Nurture Your Spiritual Self. U.S. News & World Report. 2016 Mar. https://health.usnews.com/health-news/blogs/eat-run/articles/2016-03-14/how-to-nurture-your-spiritual-self. Accessed April 20, 2020.

[255]Dresdale R. Are You Burnt Out? 10 Questions to Ask Yourself. Forbes. 2017 Aug. https://www.forbes.com/sites/rachelritlop/2017/08/03/are-you-burnt-out-10-questions-to-ask-yourself/#2c79da5f1d47. Accessed April 20, 2020.

[256]Shambaugh R. Are Chore Wars at Home Holding You Back at Work? Harvard Business Review. 2017 Jan. https://hbr.org/2017/01/are-chore-wars-at-home-holding-you-back-at- work. Accessed April 20, 2020.

[257]Smith J. A Self-Made Millionaire Says These are the 4 Things you Should do Once you Achieve Success. Business Insider. 2015 Aug. https://www.businessinsider.com/millionaire- explains-what-to-do-after-you-become-successful-2015-8. Accessed April 20, 2020.

[258]McQuilkin H, Chakrabarti M. Part IV: Are We Living in a Post-Truth World? On Point. 2020 Feb. https://www.wbur.org/onpoint/2020/02/27/part-iv-post-truth. Accessed April 20, 2020.

[259]Callinan A. Master the Concept of Leverage to Get What You Want in Business and Life. Entrepreneur. 2015 Feb. https://www.entrepreneur.com/article/242813. Accessed April 21, 2020.

[260]Cutrona CE, Wallace G, Wesner KA. Neighborhood Characteristics and Depression: An Examination of Stress Processes. Current Directions in Psychological Science: PubMed. 2006 Aug; 15(4):188-192. https://pubmed.ncbi.nlm.nih.gov/18185846/. Accessed April 20, 2020.

[261]Toren M. 3 Ways Owning Your Mistakes Will Make You Powerful. Entrepreneur. 2014 Mar. https://www.entrepreneur.com/article/232417. Accessed April 20, 2020.

[262]Gillet A, Hammond A, Martala M. Reflection: What Is It and Why Is It Useful? IAD – Institute for Academic Development. 2009. http://www.docs.hss.ed.ac.uk/iad/Learning_ teaching/Academic_pastoral/Reflect/Reflection_explanation_HO.pdf. Accessed April 20, 2020.

[263]Martin G. The Meaning and Origin of the Expression: Less is More. The Phrase Finder. 2020. https://www.phrases.org.uk/meanings/less-is-more.html. Accessed April 21, 2020.

[264]Brodt S, Six J, Feenstra G, Ingles C, Campbell D. Sustainable Agriculture. The Nature Education – Knowledge Project. 2011. https://www.nature.com/scitable/knowledge/library/sustainable-agriculture-23562787/. Accessed April 21, 2020.

[265]Leach N. How Workplace Cliques Harm the Work Environment. Alliance Work Partners. 2019 July. https://www.awpnow.com/main/2019/07/16/how-workplace-cliques-harm-the- work-environment/. Accessed April 21, 2020.

[266]Beaumont A. Why Hurrying Up Will Slow You Down. Psychology Today. 2016 June. https://www.psychologytoday.com/us/blog/handy-hints-humans/201606/why-hurrying-will- slow-you-down. Accessed April 20, 2020.

[267]Chin A. Different Generations Remembering 9/11. WSTM. 2019 Sep. https://cnycentral.com/ news/local/different-generations-remembering-911. Accessed April 21, 2020.

[268]Stöppler MC, Marks J. Home and Family: Tips for a Healthy Home Environment. MedicineNet. 2018 June. https://www.medicinenet.com/home_and_family/views.htm. Accessed April 22, 2020.

[269]Dinerstein C. Out of an Abundance of Caution, Cautiously Interpreted. American Council on Science and Health. 2017 July. https://www.acsh.org/news/2017/07/06/out-abundance- caution-cautiously-interpreted-11519. Accessed April 22, 2020.

[270]Read B. An Abundance of Caution. The Cut. 2020 Mar. https://www.thecut.com/2020/03/coronavirus-abundance-of-caution-ubiquitous.html. Accessed April 22, 2020.

[271]Sarkis SM. Preventing Social Media Burnout. Psychology Today. 2018 Sep. https://www.psychologytoday.com/us/blog/here-there-and-everywhere/201809/preventing-social-media-burnout. Accessed April 22, 2020.

[272]Gentry W. Derailment: How Successful Leaders Avoid It. Main. 2018 June. https://www.td. org/newsletters/atd-links/derailment-how-successful-leaders-avoid-it#gsc.tab=0. Accessed April 22, 2020.

[273]Henning, Ruiz & Singh. Harassment is a Factor in Workplace Burnout. HRS. 2019 June. https://www.employmentattorneyla.com/blog/2019/june/harassment-is-a-factor-in-workplace- burnout/. Accessed April 23, 2020.

[274]Brooks AW, Dai H, Schweitzer ME. I'm Sorry About the Rain! Superfluous Apologies Demonstrate Empathetic Concern and Increase Trust. Social Psychological and Personality Science. 2013; 5(4):467-474. https://www.hbs.edu/faculty/Publication%20Files/Brooks%20 Dai%20Schweitzer%202013_d2f61dc9-ec1b-485d-a815-2cf25746de50.pdf. Accessed April 23, 2020.

[275]UNC Healthcare. The Daily/Weekly Huddle: UNC Healthcare. 2010 Jan. https://news.unc healthcare.org/empnews/huddles/2010/jan18. Accessed April 24, 2020.

[276]Edwards S. Dancing and the Brain. Neurobiology – Harvard Medical School. 2020. https://neuro.hms.harvard.edu/harvard-mahoney-neuroscience-institute/brain-newsletter/and- brain/dancing-and-brain. Accessed April 25, 2020.

[277]Fuller RB. "Never Forget." PassItOn. 0AD. https://www.passiton.com/inspirational-quotes/7094-never-forget-that-you-are-one-of-a-kind-never. Accessed April 25, 2020.

[278]Thaik C. A Joyful Life Supports Good Health. HuffPost. 2014 Mar. https://www.huffpost.com/entry/joy-health_b_4612156. Accessed April 25, 2020.

[279]Ballard T. Operation Underground Railroad. OUR Rescue. 0AD. https://ourrescue.org/about#ugr. Accessed April 25, 2020.

[280]National Human Trafficking Hotline. 0AD. https://humantraffickinghotline.org/. Accessed April 25, 2020.

[281]Yi H, Carrel P, Martin M, et al. Shaping the Future of Economic Progress. World Economic Forum. 2020. https://www.weforum.org/platforms/shaping-the-future-of-the-new-economy- and-society. Accessed April 25, 2020.

[282]Stephens S. What's Keeping You from Going Further? Becoming Minimalist. 2019 Sep. https://www.becomingminimalist.com/go-further/. Accessed April 25, 2020.

[283]Razzetti G. Forgiving is Hard, but Not Forgiving Hurts More. Liberationist. 2019 Oct. https://liberationist.org/forgiving-is-hard-but-not-forgiving-hurts-more/. Accessed April 25, 2020.

[284]Jeffrey S. A Definitive Guide to Self-Actualization (Based on Maslow's Findings). CEOSage. 2020 Feb. https://scottjeffrey.com/self-actualization/. Accessed April 25, 2020.

[285]Carmen A. Seeing the Bigger Picture: Life Maybe Better Than You Think - How a New Perspective Can Create More Joy in your Life. Psychology Today. 2015 Jan. https://www. psychologytoday.com/hk/blog/the-gift-maybe/201501/seeing-the-bigger-picture-life-maybe- better-you-think. Accessed April 25, 2020.

[286]AAI. Why Climb Mountains? American Alpine Institute – Courses, Ascents, Expeditions. 2018. https://www.alpineinstitute.com/get-started/why-climb-mountains. Accessed April 25, 2020.

[287]Burkus D. Why Climbing the Corporate Ladder May Be the Worst Path to the Top. Quartz at Work. 2018 July. https://qz.com/work/1335172/why-climbing-the-corporate-ladder-may-be- the-worst-path-to-the-top/. Accessed April 25, 2020.

[288]Phoenix S. 4 Reasons Why Millennials Don't Want to Climb the Corporate Ladder. Medium. 2017 Jan. https://medium.com/@stevenphoenix/4-reasons-why-millennials-dont-want-to- climb-the-corporate-ladder-e951c35fb35b. Accessed April 25, 2020.

[289]Rucker M. Why You Need More Fun in Your Life, According to Science. Michael Rucker, Ph.D. 2016 Dec. https://michaelrucker.com/having-fun/why-you-need-more-fun-in-your-life/. Accessed April 25, 2020.

[290]Hayley. How to Make Meaningful Connections in a Modern World. Nourished Planner. 2018 Feb. https://nourishedplanner.com/meaningful-connections/. Accessed April 25, 2020.

[291]Chaffee T. How to Make Meaningful Connections. Fortune. 2016 Apr. https://fortune.com/2016/04/11/how-to-make-meaningful-connections/. Accessed April 25, 2020.

[292]Hunter WC. Liars. In: Ginger Snaps; a Book of Business Helps. Kansas City, MO: Hunter Service; (1915):103.

[293]Pfiffner J. Trump's Lies Corrode Democracy. Brookings Institution. 2018 Apr. https://www. brookings.edu/blog/fixgov/2018/04/13/trumps-lies-corrode-democracy/. Accessed April 25, 2020.

[294]Ronsoak. The Lies and Lack of Self Respect that Lead to Burnout. DEV Community. 2019 May. https://dev.to/ronsoak/the-lies-and-lack-of-self-respect-that-lead-to-burnout-5007. Accessed April 25, 2020.

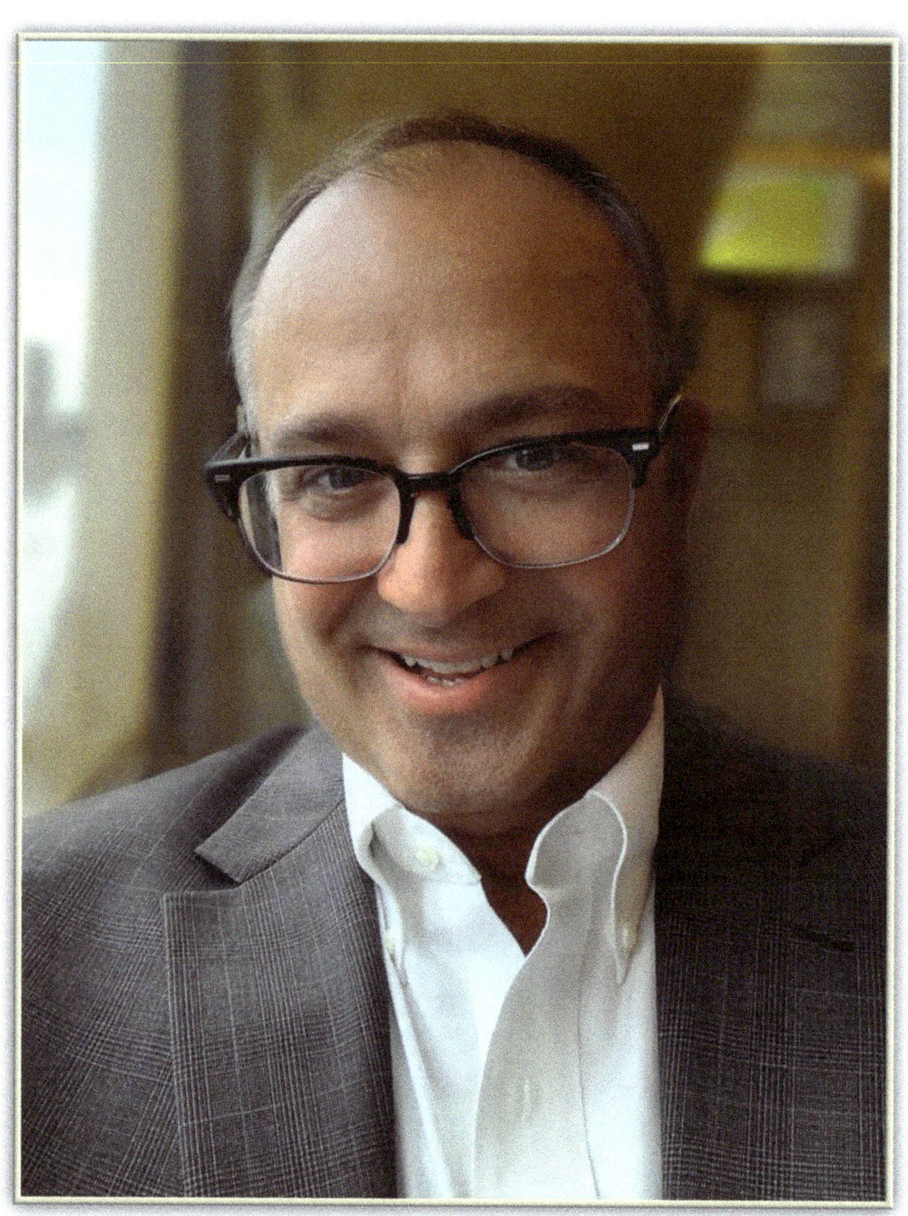

About the Author

Dr. Richard C. Scepura possesses strong credentials as a successful Nurse Executive. He is certified by American Nurses Credentialing Center as an Advanced Board-Certified Nurse Executive. He is also certified by the Nephrology Nursing Certification Commission as a Certified Dialysis Nurse. Richard has consulted and directed for *Seattle Children's Hospital, Steward Healthcare/St. Elizabeth's Medical Center* in Boston, MA, and managed for UNC Healthcare in Chapel Hill, NC. He began his career at *Beth Israel Deaconess Medical Center* (a Harvard teaching hospital) while living in the North End of Boston, MA, in the 1990s. He graduated from the University of Massachusetts with a double major Baccalaureate of Science in Psychology and Nursing. After several years as a staff RN, Richard began an exciting travel nurse career. He practiced in 14 U.S. states over a decade, working mostly in world-class magnet healthcare facilities across the nation serving different populations.

While working for UNC Hospitals, he attended Pfeiffer University in Research Triangle Park, NC, and received his joint degree, the MBA/MHA, Magna Cum Laude concentrating on Leadership and Change Management. His doctorate is in Nursing Practice (DNP) from Clarion and Edinboro Universities of Pennsylvania, graduating Summa Cum Laude. His doctoral project is titled, "*Intending to Stay - Retention, Burnout, Structural Empowerment and Dialysis Nursing: Integrating Kanter's Theory and the Refined Nurse Worklife Model*" and the abstract was selected for presentation at the American Nephrology Nursing Association National Symposium in May, 2021. He also published an article for the American Organization of Nurse Leaders in the *Nurse Leader* academic journal titled, "*The Challenges with Pre-Employment Testing and the Potential for Hiring Bias.*" He is a volunteer editorial board member for The American Journal of Management Science and Engineering as well as an editorial reviewer for MDPI: Nursing Reports Quarterly. Now, he brings to his colleagues, or any reader in need, in the most serious times of peril with Covid-19, the light-hearted thoughtful book that makes you "think," *The Healing Burnout Guide.*

Author's Note

A Special Thank You to the Artists- Without your talent, the self-reflection journals wouldn't be as purposeful. We appreciate your thoughtfulness and contributions in this great effort. We hope you enjoy the series and are sincerely pleased to promote your creations.

Artist Courtesy Credit List

Berkise, Edward	edward.berkise@gmail.com
Brown, Rachel	www.rachel-e-brown.com/Work t
Chisholm, Jon	craigchism@twc.com
DelMonte, Barbara	barbaradelmonte2@gmail.com
Dunne, Kevin	kdunnek@gmail.com
Ensign, Nancy Nixon	nancynixonensign@gmail.com
French, Christine	christinefrench@me.com
Gonzalez, Maika	www.artmajeur.com/artedemaika/
Grayson, Aryn	nyra1266@gmail.com
Gutierrez, Susan	susanjgutierrez@outlook.com
Hodge, Judy	jhodge@urbanmindshare.com
Holland, Robert John	dotnbob@netsync.net
Julien, Marla	silversky26@hotmail.com
Kamperveen, Umberto	umberto@umbertokamperveenart.com
Kelly, Toni	toni@tonikellystudio.com
Lafferty, Ronnie	ronnielafferty60@gmail.com
Larson, Patti	pattilarsonphotos@outlook.com
Long, Charles Freedom	charlesfreedomlong@gmail.com
MacKay, Susan	smofny@stny.rr.com
Marquis, Eduardo Andres	eamt1966@gmail.com
Mattson, Jill	jillimattson@yahoo.com
Merrins, Marcia	mmerrins@netsync.net
Parker, Ann	anna242parker@yahoo.com
Probst, Linda	mikeandlindaprobst@yahoo.com
Rubin, Mara	rubinmaraci@hotmail.com
Samler, Rebecca	beckysamler1@gmail.com
Santi, Jill	jillswriting@hotmail.com
Schultz, Lisa	lschultz18102@gmail.com
Shank, Carrie	tothetopcj@gmail.com
Smith, Bill	Lorencsmith@twlakes.net
Spar Ki	sparki3114@icloud.com
Turner, Peter S.	psterlingtri@gmail.com

Contributors

Contributors:

Curator Nancy Nixon Ensign
Contributing Editor Tiffany Smith
Contributing Editor Jessica Olma
Graphic Designer and Publisher Tom Olson (Pixel-Pencil Studio and Morningstar Press)

The Artists of:

Barcelona, ES
Bennington, VT
Chautauqua County, NY
Erie County, NY
Erie County, PA
Gaios, GR
Manhattan, NY
Marathon, FL
Newport, RI
Toronto, CA
Woodstock, NY

Peer Reviewers:

Dr. Jane Blystone, PhD
Dr. Meg Larson, DNP

Curator and Cover Background Art

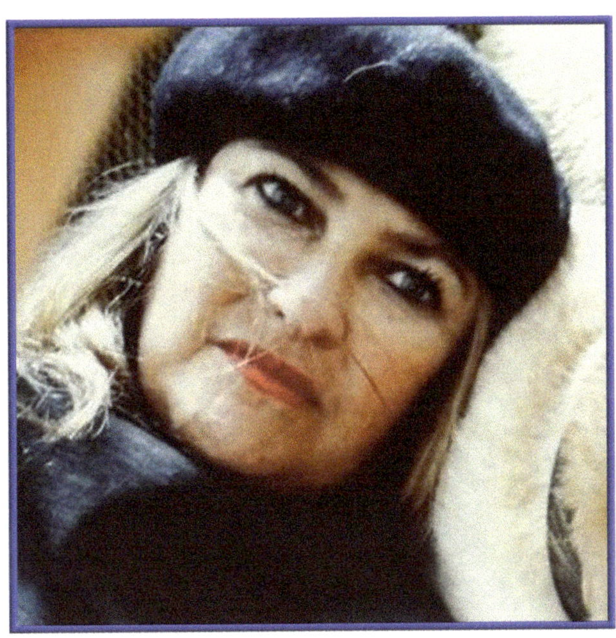

Nancy Nixon Ensign is a native Chautauqua County NY artist, third-generation maternal painter, and great-grandniece to impressionist *Edward Willis Redfield.* After graduating from *Rochester Institute of Technology* (RIT), she moved to Cleveland, OH, advancing her skills in ceramic and glass jewelry design while living at the *Hodge School Studios and Galleries.* Years later, Nancy moved to NYC to work as a set designer for *Victor Scenic* while also studying Byzantine Iconography at the *School of Sacred Arts.*

To escape winter, Nancy moved to Orlando, FL, and worked as a scenic artist for *Walt Disney World and Universal Studios.* Ten years later, she returned to Chautauqua County and was offered the position of *Patterson Library Octagon Gallery* Curator, installing well over 200 exhibitions. Currently, Nancy is Vice President and Exhibition Chair for the *North Shore Arts Alliance*, which she and seven other artists formed in 2008. Nancy and her husband, Jake, reside in Western New York, where she creates artwork in her home studio. *"I feel blessed and grateful to participate as curator, confidant, and friend to Richard."*

Contributing Editor

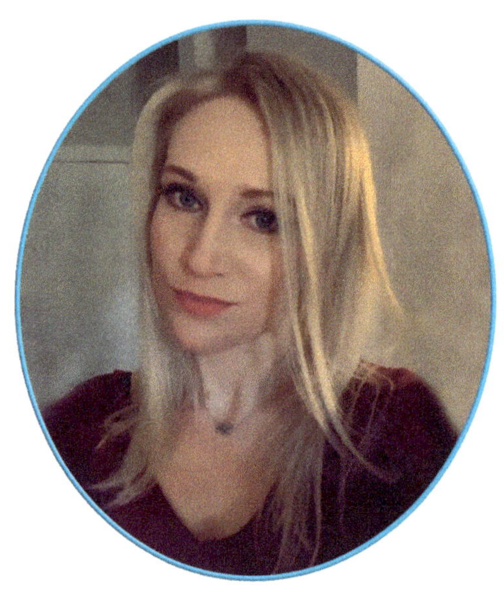

Tiffany Lynn Smith is a native of *Chautauqua County, NY*. After graduating from *Jamestown Community College* with an associate degree in Business Administration, she moved to Tempe, AZ, to continue her education at *Arizona State University (ASU).* There, Tiffany studied and graduated with a BA in English Literature with a focus on Business and Professional Writing/Editing. In Arizona, she worked as a technical writer for Kizen Group, an ASU eSeed Venture.

Tiffany then moved to Charlotte, NC, where she currently resides. She has held management positions in both the service industry and retail, most recently for *Michael Kors*. She now works as an office administrator/medical assistant for *Lake Norman Integrative Wellness*. Tiffany is very passionate about technical writing and provides contractual editing services.

Contributing Editor

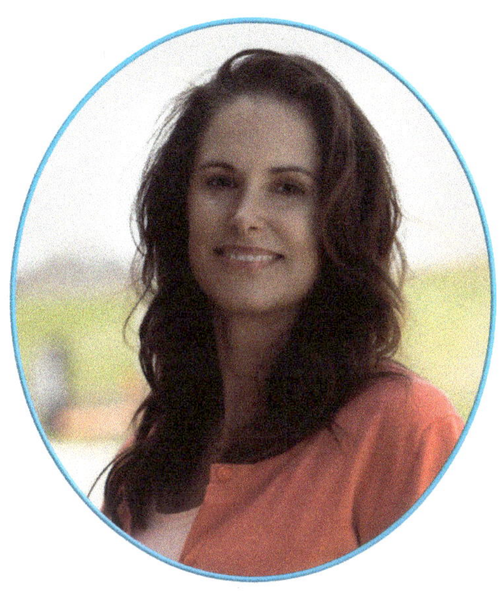

Jessica Olma is a writer and editor. Originally from Vancouver, BC, Canada, she obtained dual citizenship in the US and moved throughout the country, settling in North Coventry, PA, where she attended college at Temple University's Elkins Park Art Campus. In 2014, after raising her family, she attended Colorado Technical University to pursue her passion for writing and editing. Jessica established *Scribe Syndicate* in Charlotte, NC, to offer writing and editing services to various clients who publish information in print and online. As the business grew, she moved to Denver, CO, and collaborates nationally on digital marketing projects. Jessica works closely with publishers, authors, web designers, marketing consultants, and business owners to write and edit eBooks, web page copy, blog articles, white papers, and more. She ensures her clients are seen as experts in their field who provide high-quality information and education to the public and consumers. She is honored to be part of Dr. Richard Scepura's book, *The Healing Burnout Guide.*

Graphic Designer and Publisher

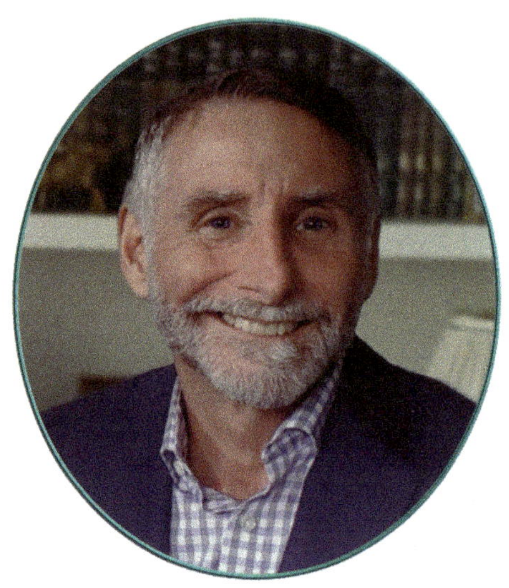

Tom Olson is the founder of Pixel-Pencil Studio, a graphic design agency in Rye, NY specializing in publications. With more than 20 years of Manhattan agency experience, Tom places the highest priority on superior client service, creativity and attention to detail.

Tom also leads Morningstar Press, a publishing service for independent authors, providing a comprehensive and flexible array of services for authors to tap as needed to take their book project from the idea phase to a virtual book launch.

https://PixelPencilStudio.com

https://www.Morningstar.Press

SEASON THREE

Proficient

My Hobbies

Patience

Practice Makes Perfect

Independence

Not Getting What You Want

An Olive Branch

Recognition

Prudence

Economic Insecurity

Life Isn't Always Easy

Feeling Appreciated

Stop Worrying

I'm Worth It

Pay and Economics

Sharing Your Stories

Pushy People and Agendas

Elder Care and Working

Overcommitting

Spending Time

Misconduct

Divisions

Being Relevant

Harmony

Setting Boundaries

Working Parents

Generations at Work

Taking a ME Day

Meditation and Mindfulness

Looking Out the Window

Personal Boundaries

Avoid Gossip

Having PEP

Doubting Yourself

Grit

Privacy

Being Cooperative

Setting New SMART Goals

Civility

Social Justice

Growing from Mistakes

Verbal Abuse at Work

Making a Wish

Terminated

Having Your Back

Concentrating on the Positive

Popularity

Drawing the Line

Being Nimble

Certain Expectations

Is Human Resources Your Friend?

Labeling People

Think

Pandemic Traumatic Stress

Getting the Experience

Sound Judgment

Quitting

Progress and AI

Relaxing your Mind

Your Critical Inner Voice

Nurturing Your Spirit

Getting Enough Sleep

Chore Wars

Achieving

Misinformation

Leveraging

The Neighborhood

Being Reasonable

Reflecting

Less is More

Banding Together

Cliques at Work

Faster, Hurry

Remembrance

My Home Environment

Abundance of Caution

Social Media and Burnout

Derailment

Equal Opportunity

Apologizing

Dancing

I'm One of a Kind

Living Joy

Being Rescued

Shaping the Future

Go Further than Before

Forgiving

Actualizing

The Bigger Picture

Climbing

Having Some Fun

Meaningful Connections

Don't Lie to Me

www.ingramcontent.com/pod-product-compliance
Ingram Content Group UK Ltd.
Pitfield, Milton Keynes, MK11 3LW, UK
UKHW061955290726
14090UKWH00021B/1236